Cautionary Tales

Authentic Case Histories
from Medical Practice

Cautionary Tales

Authentic Case Histories from Medical Practice

John Murtagh AO

MBBS, MD, BSc, BEd, FRACGP, DipObstRCOG
Emeritus Professor in General Practice, School of Primary Health Care,
Monash University Melbourne, Victoria
Professorial Fellow, Department of General Practice, University of
Melbourne, Victoria
Adjunct Clinical Professor, Graduate School of Medicine, University of Notre
Dame, Fremantle, Western Australia

Sara Bird

MBBS, MFM (Clin), FRACGP
Executive Manager, MDA National Insurance Pty Ltd

This third edition published 2019
First edition published 1992, second edition published 2011
Text © 2019 John Murtagh and Sara Bird
Illustrations and design © 2019 McGraw-Hill Education (Australia) Pty Ltd

National Library of Australia Cataloguing-in-Publication Data:

A catalogue record for this book is available from the National Library of Australia

Author: John Murtagh, Sara Bird
Title: Cautionary Tales
Edition: 3rd edition
ISBN: 9781743767443

Published in Australia by
McGraw-Hill Education (Australia) Pty Ltd
Level 33, 680 George Street, Sydney NSW 2000
Publisher: Diane Gee-Clough
Production editor: Lara McMurray
Copyeditor: Yani Silvana
Proofreader: Lindsey Langston
Cover design: Christa Moffitt, christabella designs
Cover image: Photographee.eu/Shutterstock
Internal design: SPi, India
Author photograph: Gerrit Fokkema Photography
Original illustrations: Diane Booth
Typeset in STIX MathJax Main 10/14 by SPi, India
Printed in China on 80 gsm woodfree by 1010 Printing Int. Ltd

Foreword

Problem-based learning is now established as the preferred method in clinical medicine. Although our own medical education may have led us to believe that a solid base of theoretical knowledge was needed on which to build our clinical knowledge, the evidence of the past 50 years supports the view that we learn best by doing, by experiencing real-life situations, either personally or vicariously through case histories. There is nothing new or startling about this. All this century and well before it, educators have been saying this and lamenting the relative paucity of problem-based learning in schools and universities.

In the first two editions of *Cautionary Tales,* John Murtagh provided a rich collection of case histories, which medical educators at both graduate and undergraduate levels have found invaluable in teaching and learning. These case histories are all the more valuable because they are enriched with the psychosocial elements that form part of almost every patient problem and every transaction between the patient and the doctor. Indeed, these elements are so central that to ignore them in favour of the purely physical is to often miss the point altogether. Medicine is still inclined to embrace the biomedical model, to which can be attributed countless advances in medicine during this century. But there are many phenomena that this limited model is unable to explain. An expanded biomedical model that weaves the web of psychological, social and environmental factors into the biomedical warp, serves us and our patients much better. *Cautionary Tales* provides many of the examples we need to illustrate this expanded model.

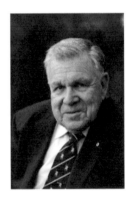

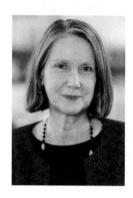

This considerably revised third edition has been enhanced by the addition of Dr Sara Bird as John's co-author. Sara, who has an experienced background in general practice in Sydney, has added a significant complement of real-life cases that she has encountered in her experience as Manager Medico-legal and Advisory Services, MDA National. Over the past 20 years, Sara has worked in the role of assisting general practitioners and their staff in dealing with a variety of medico-legal issues which arise in general practice, including medical negligence claims, complaints, Coronial enquiries and other investigations. She is also the author of the *Medico-legal Handbook for General Practice*. Sara provides an expert commentary on the previous and new case histories.

The addition of the feature 'Discussion and lessons learned' to each tale, the use of the questioning format and Sara's medico-legal commentary, further enhances the value of the tales. Drawn mostly from Professor Murtagh's own practice in rural Victoria, where literally anything can and often does happen, they have an authenticity that the artificially created case history can never match.

Educators will find *Cautionary Tales* a source of excellent material for teaching and learning, and learners too will derive from them pleasure, insight, and wisdom as well.

W. E. Fabb, AM, FRACGP, FRCGP

Foundation National Director of Education,
Family Medicine Programme, Australia
Past Professor of Family Medicine, Chinese University of Hong Kong
Past CEO, World Organisation of Family Doctors (Wonca)

Contents

Preface

To practise medicine is a privilege, to practise it well is a difficult challenge, but not to learn from one's mistakes is unforgivable.

Cautionary Tales is a collection of authentic case histories encountered over 50 years of practising medicine, especially by John Murtagh and his wife, Jill Rosenblatt, during 10 years of intense yet wonderful, general practice in a country area of Victoria, Australia. It was their privilege to be the sole practitioners to a hard-working farming community of 2700 people. The practice was located in a small township with a twelve-bed Bush Nursing Hospital. The area, which was mountainous bushland with a snow resort, was popular with tourists. Many of the tales pertain to the experience of knowing their patients so well—both professionally and personally. They reflect the intensely human side of our calling and to share them is a special privilege. It is also appropriate to ponder on the humorous side of some of our experiences as well as the inevitable tragic outcomes for so many that we remember with sadness.

The concept of, and impetus for producing, a series of cautionary tales followed the obvious fascination of my medical students who considered they learned so much from them, especially when they realised they really happened and were certainly not apocryphal, however embellished in presentation.

Experience for doctors comes from the stories of our patients and, at times, our colleagues. As doctors, we are challenged by the atypical presentation of a common disease and the typical presentation of a rare disease. Each of the case histories in this book is a cautionary tale from which we can learn and observe the humanity of general practice.

We hope that sharing our experiences and messages is an important contribution to continuing medical education. In particular, the cautionary advice about so many pitfalls is extremely useful to the inexperienced doctor facing up to the vast challenge of general practice. There has been a focus on the medico-legal dimension of the tales, so that we can develop a healthy awareness of the pitfalls of our shortcomings, especially the missed diagnosis. This medico-legal commentary has been enhanced by the co-authorship of Sara Bird, who brings her special expertise and understanding to the editorial. Sara has also provided authentic case histories from her experience in medico-legal practice. We believe that the subject matter covered in this book is a reasonably accurate reflection of the common traps facing doctors in Western medicine. The tales are presented under headings that capture the nature of the message. Authoritative commentary on relevant medico-legal advice and pitfalls is provided using the case histories as a platform. The book concludes with an overview of a strategy that may help to keep the margin of diagnostic error to a minimum.

Good judgement is based on experience. Experience is based on poor judgement.

We trust that our shared experiences promote a certain wisdom, insight and better judgement.

Acknowledgments

The authors would like to acknowledge the support of the Royal Australian College of General Practitioners in encouraging the concept of *Cautionary Tales* and for their permission to reproduce material that has appeared in *Australian Family Physician.* We also acknowledge the many practitioners who have supported the series through individual contributions or through popular support.

Individual contributions to this book have come from the following general practitioners to whom we are indebted:

Peter Baquie:	Doctor, watch your words; Tales of *Campylobacter jejuni*
Karen Barry:	Beware the sweats by night
Frank M. Cave:	A shock to the system; Diabetes with a difference
Jim Colquhoun:	The concealment enigma: why is it so?; The widow's rejection; Lame duck survival; The ticket of entry; Missing links; Not an easy game; Alive, well and not to be forgotten; 'Sacked'; A certain kind of madness; An unkindness of cancers
Brian Connor:	Decisions, decisions in the elderly
Dr Sheila Cronin:	The lovelorn patient
Trish Dunning:	Insulin stopwork
Chris Fogarty:	Saga 1: Hot flushes (in 'Alcoholics anonymous')
Andrew Fraser:	She was, of course, a doctor's wife; Home visits: three cautionary tales; A doctor's 'heartburn'; Don't work in the dark!
Peter Graham:	No lead in his pencil
Wadie Haddad:	Pyrexia in an Asian migrant; Chest pain of unusual cause
Wayne Herdy:	An unusual presentation of a common disorder

Christopher Hill:	Careful what you say!; Glimpses of a cruel world
Don Lewis:	Sidetracked
Lance Le Ray:	Some 'sort of vascular phenomenon'
Donna Mak:	Marital surprises
Hugo Matthews:	A super mimic
Breck McKay:	Thoroughly analysing Milly; Fits and funny turns: the case of Terryanne
Amanda Nutting:	Paper-clip problems
Anthony Palmer:	Summer and *pseudomonas*
Andrew Patrick:	A real headache
Leon Piterman:	Big-headed and pig-headed; IUDs and ectopic pregnancy
Geoff Quail:	Oh for a suntan!
Philip Ridge:	Beware children and needle-sticks
Ralph Sacks:	A bronze medal
Lyn Scoles:	Slowing up: it's just old age . . . or is it?
Leslie Segal:	Keeping a stiff upper lip
Chris Silagy:	The high-spirited schoolteacher
Roger Smith:	Keeping an open mind
Gino Toncich:	Case 1: The child who 'died' (in 'Two "fishy" tales')
Alan Tucker:	The prescription pad
Bill Walker:	Twin trouble
Alan Watson:	Are you playing Russian roulette with your patients?

A NOTE TO READERS

Many of the tales in this book have cryptic headings so that the diagnosis is not apparent. You are invited to analyse the case history and study the clinical findings and the minimal information to make a provisional diagnosis prior to reading the part describing the diagnosis and outcome. All of these cases are authentic, but the names have been altered.

Embarrassing moments

Black spot

We were very busy with sick patients, teaching students and the GP registrar, and taking many phone calls. However, I stopped to answer a query from our registrar who was inspecting a very black lesion on the forearm of a middle-aged male patient: 'Do you think I should excise this suspicious pigmented lesion?' After a cursory glance I said, 'A good idea—use the standard elliptical excision with a 3 mm margin and send it to pathology'.

A few days later the bemused registrar showed me the report—'black paint'. Yes, indeed it was and the patient, now supporting an unnecessary wound, confirmed that he had been painting in the days preceding the consultation. We had both learned a valuable lesson—take a good history, don't rush decisions and be very careful when you are extra busy and stressed. It would be best practice to acquire a dermatoscope and become skilled in its use.

Smart alec prognostications

I had just commenced country practice and was trying hard to create a good impression with the locals, who were certainly curious to assess their new doctor from the fledgling Monash Medical School. One of the district's matriarchs brought her 66-year-old sister who was visiting from Melbourne for a check-up. The consultation was pleasantly social, with no actual presenting problem and all aspects of the history were normal, as was the physical examination. In particular the cardiovascular examination, including the pulse and blood pressure, was normal. I informed her that on my examination she was in good health and could look forward to the immediate future. Unfortunately she died suddenly two days later from a cerebrovascular accident.

This episode, which must have set people talking in a small rural community, was a real lesson that one can never be too smug with medical prognostications. This was about the time I started to produce education leaflets for my patients.

With friends like these . . .

Gloria was the effervescent catering manager at the major hospital where I ran the staff clinic part-time. Born in London, she was a great character who was full of banter, noise and mischief. She was a regular attendee with multiple minor problems and she joked that her reason for attending was that she was fond of the doctor! One evening there was a huge function at the hospital where the guests included dignitaries such as federal and state politicians, hospital administrators, senior university management and senior consultants. As I walked into the hall I saw Gloria, the hostess, all dressed up and looking like I'd never seen her before. Then from the other side of the hall in the loudest possible voice came the shocker, 'What's up, John? Don't you recognise me with my clothes on?' What could one say?

Wrong injection, wrong person

The next embarrassing experience could hardly have been worse, especially as the patient was a lawyer. New to the practice, he presented with severe shoulder pain caused by subacromial bursitis. We treated it with a local injection of 'Depo-Medrol' and Xylocaine. However, I noticed later that the ampoule read Depo-Provera and that the ampoules of Depo-Provera and Depo-Medrol looked almost identical. I decided that it was important to contact him and admit the mistake and provide information on ancillary measures to help recovery of the problem. He was very reasonable about the mistake and fortunately his shoulder predictably settled.

The lesson to us was to check and double-check all drugs—especially injectable drugs—meticulously, particularly as our relatively small practice did not have the advantage of a practice nurse.

Blood donor to recipient in four days

Helen, a 27-year-old farmer, presented with a breast lump 3–4 cm in diameter. Clinically and on imaging it seemed benign. A fine needle aspiration biopsy indicated fibroadenoma. Helen was keen to have the lump excised. It happened that she came to our blood donation service three days before elective surgery to excise the lump. She joked that she might need it later but I scoffed at the thought, saying that I had never had a bleeding problem with breast surgery. However, she had a reactionary haemorrhage some hours after the procedure, lost a substantial amount of blood and required a transfusion. One of the bottles used was Helen's very own blood.

Oops—wrong bedroom!

The following account is described by our colleague Dr David Game AO (Game, 1990) who practised in a very fashionable Adelaide suburb.

When I am called out at night I always request that the front veranda light is put on as this aids the identification of the house in a dark street in the middle of the night. While doing one particular late night call, I noticed a veranda light on in the street and thought that I had arrived at my destination.

My knock on the door was answered by a rather startled man in his dressing gown. I promptly said 'Good evening', walked straight in, past the startled man, down the hall to the bedroom and stood by the bed looking down at an equally startled lady. It was to my horror that I realised that I had entered the wrong house.

I tried to make my apologies and excuses as I backed out of the house, expecting to be assaulted or at least abused by the husband. However, he simply said, 'Don't worry Doctor, but I can tell you one thing. I have never seen a man get into a woman's bedroom as quickly as you can'.

Caught out by the law

Mrs N, an ex-nurse, rang me to say that she was concerned about her 17-year-old son Eric, who had abdominal pain and diarrhoea. Shortly after, I noticed Eric walking with difficulty, limping along the footpath to the surgery, bent forwards, holding his lower abdomen and looking very pale. I said to his mother 'Looks like a ruptured appendix'. Well, the spot diagnosis was correct and he actually had an appendiceal abscess but all went well with the operation. Mrs N was very complimentary.

Post-operative ward visits to the phlegmatic young man were interesting. He was extremely shy, courteous, tough, resilient and non-complaining. He expressed a desire to become a surgeon.

Nine years later I was returning home from a conference in Canberra and to my shame was caught speeding on the Hume Highway. To my surprise the magistrate at Wangaratta suspended my licence for one month. I had to report to the Malvern police station to hand in my licence to none other than a bemused Constable Eric N. After 31 days of difficulty hitching rides and riding bikes, I fronted the still quietly spoken but tough policeman to retrieve my driver's licence. Apart from the coincidence and embarrassment this was a real cautionary tale about responsible road behaviour and a reminder that doctors get no special favours even for a one-off offence. I had blotted my copy-book with my phlegmatic ex-patient. And Mrs N had the last word: 'You're not so clever after all'.

A forgotten home visit

One day I was walking along our small shopping strip and noticed Mrs Stafford, a pleasant middle-aged lady, who suffered from trigeminal neuralgia that occasionally required strong analgesia. To my dismay I realised that she had recently called me in the middle of the night requesting a home visit and it didn't eventuate. I asked, 'Was I dreaming, or did you ring me the other night?'

'Yes, I did and I rang back and you were engaged. The pain settled and I didn't bother you again.' I could visualise myself sound asleep (after a heavy night delivering babies) still holding the phone. It was the second occurrence (I think!) so from then on, I made certain to switch on the radio as soon as I received a night call.

Who's Bill?

On another occasion I received a middle-of-night distress call from a woman who sounded quite hysterical. 'John—come quickly—it's Bill—he's collapsed—it's urgent!' Then silence. I sat on the edge of the bed in a quandary thinking 'Who on earth is Bill?' I really had no idea and waited for inspiration or a further call. After a long hour or so the phone rang. 'John, you haven't popped in yet—what's going on?' 'Where do I pop?' I asked. She identified herself and to my surprise it was a young man who lived only 100 m away. I arrived to find Bill sitting up in bed looking fit and healthy. I determined that it was an episode of micturition syncope on top of a heavy drinking bout the previous evening. The lesson of course is to get precise details despite the somnolent haze.

Unexpected obstructions, including dead people

In a country practice without a local ambulance service, the use of a car with emergency equipment on board is essential. My garage was behind the juxtaposed surgery and residence with the driveway beside the surgery. One night I was called to the hospital but only managed 100 m—no petrol—the tank had again been drained—a special lock was required.

One morning I went to attend an obstetric case only to discover that a huge heap of screenings (to service the driveway) had been dumped at the top of the drive next to the garage. Furious shovelling followed.

On another occasion I found a car in the driveway with a dead unknown person inside. He had had severe back pain and felt extremely unwell and had decided on recommendation to drive 120 km to see me. Post mortem revealed that the poor fellow had a ruptured aortic aneurysm. Sadly we occasionally found dead or collapsed people at the door of the surgery or residence or sitting outside in a car.

We did not have an appointment system during the day and people would just turn up. Once I noticed a person sitting quietly in a corner of the waiting room at the end of the day and upon checking him found that he was dead. The upset relatives said, 'What did you do to him?' We eventually used an appointment system.

Another incident occurred in our staff clinic when a man with a Box Hill identity came for assessment of long-standing low back pain. When I saw him I could not assess his back because he had neurological symptoms in his arm and leg. It was due to the unfortunate coincidence of a stroke in evolution. When I contacted his work the upsetting response 'What did you do to him?' was echoed. General practice can be tough at times.

An uninteresting problem!

I had just completed a long 'shopping list' consultation with one of my 'heartsink' patients and slipped out the back to check on the progress of an extension to the practice, when the patient walked by with her husband. 'I don't think he's interested in my problem at all', I overheard the elderly Mrs E say.

This comment pulled me up with a shock as I took pride in being interested and caring about my patients and every problem. When I mused over the consultation I realised that it was the last problem of unsatisfactory defecation that I had not paid much attention to. She was absolutely correct. (I'd been listening to a litany of elimination problems all morning during my hospital and nursing home rounds!)

Chastised I decided to contact her and say that I was concerned about a couple of her problems and would like to review her. Mrs E was bemused but delighted. She did in fact have a rectal prolapse and she must have wondered why she received such devoted attention, including surgery by a surgical colleague. The lesson is to treat all problems as serious and perhaps it would be salutary for us to be a 'fly on the wall' and hear what our patients really think of the quality of their care.

'Are you trying to kill me, Doc?'

Derek, a 42-year-old English teacher, was a great English character with the adult version of ADHD. I had performed a haemorrhoidectomy on him and was reviewing him in hospital the following morning. He was uncharacteristically subdued and looked dreadful—a pale, sickly green hue like one of the Four Horsemen of the Apocalypse (Death!). I felt uneasy as I thought he must be bleeding from somewhere. 'Are you trying to poison me, Doc?' he said. 'Do I really have to eat all that dreadful stuff?'

I then noticed a great lump of about 50–70 g of Vegemite in a specimen bottle. The fiendish nurse had told him 'Doc Murtagh thinks it's great medicine, especially for expats!' Vegemite was off the breakfast menu thenceforth, except if requested.

Better out than Ricky Ponting!

At times the very human function of passing flatus can cause embarrassment for a patient, especially in this era of taking lipid-lowering agents. Our professional responsibility is to remain stoic and indifferent should it occur in our presence. Some years ago a young lad of about nineteen was getting off the couch when he passed wind with considerable sound effect. Without any change in body language he looked at me and said laconically, 'Better out than Allan Border'. It was a classic spontaneous response.

On another occasion I was conducting a hospital ward round when an elderly gentleman broke wind and exclaimed casually, 'Well, Doc, better an empty house than a bad tenant'. My professional response is to ignore these incidents but if someone (usually a young male) looks at me for a reaction it is 'Better out than Ricky Ponting'.

What do you think?

The patient was a well-groomed young woman in her late twenties. One of my partners had asked me to see her because of persistent interscapular back pain. I asked her to remove some clothing but keep her underwear on. When I entered the examination room she was sitting on the couch naked to the waist preening herself in front of the mirror and rotating her torso to enhance her 'Playboy-like' chest. 'What do you think, Doctor?' she said with confidence.

I was caught off guard and felt most uneasy. My rule was to never— but never ever—pass comment about a person's anatomy, especially about any abnormality and particularly about breasts or genital organs in both sexes. Stalling for time I said, 'Why do you ask?' Then I noticed the recent pink scars of cosmetic surgery immediately inferior to the breasts. It was prudent to say, 'Perhaps you can tell me the name of your impressive surgeon'.

The asthma inhaler shemozzle

Violet, who suffered from many medical problems, presented at the age of 67 with adult-onset asthma. I was quite puzzled until I realised that her ophthalmologist had changed her eye drops to the beta-blocker timolol. She did have a history of childhood asthma. I prescribed a salbutamol inhaler and went through the demonstration of its use with a follow-up education sheet.

About two weeks later the pharmacist who was conducting her home medication review rang me. The patient had complained to the pharmacist that the medication had not helped. 'What on earth did you teach her?' he quipped mischievously. He said that it was no wonder she hadn't responded to the medication as she was using the puffer with the cap still on. I know of course that I should have taken more time to get her to demonstrate the technique to me.

A few years ago, some doctors at an asthma seminar in Melbourne were comparing the various inappropriate ways in which patients were found to use their anti-asthma aerosols. The following were recorded (believe me!):

- sprayed directly onto the chest
- sprayed under the arm
- sprayed up the nose
- sprayed onto the bed (to kill mites).

Chapter 2

Great mimics

Cupid's disease

It was in the 1960s when I first met the one truly 'mad' person that I encountered in my medical career. I had just commenced a short rotation as a psychiatric RMO at a reputable Melbourne psychiatric hospital. The patient was a 52-year-old Londoner who had migrated to Australia with her husband and son. She had been 'certified' to the hospital with the presumptive diagnosis of 'mania—for management'! Taking a history was difficult as she was forever restless, distracted and had flights of ideas. Furthermore she had an alluring 'fetching' body language, which led to sexual escapades in the hospital grounds with the inevitable willing male inpatients. She was soon accommodated in a secure ward and was assessed by the medical director and a consultant neurologist—two extremely brilliant clinicians.

As they left the ward they said, 'John, we want you to perform a lumbar puncture—we suspect neurosyphilis'. This came as a surprise in view of her apparent clean-cut background and doting family members. However, we did determine that she had probably had sexual encounters with servicemen who lived in the family boarding house during World War II.

Well, my futile attempt at performing the procedure was a nightmare which remains with me to this day. The shrieking and wailing (I kept thinking that a banshee would sound like her) were punctuated by threats to the nurse and to me of injury from the instruments we were handling. I was honestly frightened by this unfortunate woman and felt so sad that a human being could be so tormented and manic.

The boss was not impressed with my failure but I heard that the specialist team's effort to get the cerebrospinal fluid under general anaesthesia was like a scene from Dante's 'Inferno'. The spinal fluid did test positive for syphilis.

She was treated with parenteral penicillin and large doses of antipsychotics but unfortunately I have no information about the eventual outcome.

DISCUSSION AND LESSONS LEARNED

- Our patient probably had Cupid's disease, which is increased libido in older people with neurosyphilis, as described by Oliver Sacks in *The Man Who Mistook His Wife for a Hat* (Sacks, 1985).
- Fortunately tertiary syphilis is rare but we now know that primary syphilis is staging a comeback especially with associated HIV infection.
- Penicillin is most effective for primary syphilis but unlikely to be effective at the tertiary level. A particular problem with treatment by penicillin is the dramatic Jarisch–Herxheimer reaction, albeit of low morbidity. The reaction can be modified with concomitant use of oral corticosteroids (Fauci et al., 2008).
- Think twice about performing a procedure—even a simple one—on a mentally ill patient. Plan carefully.

A super mimic

The patient was a 71-year-old male, a native of Papua New Guinea, resident in Australia for six years. He presented with fever, diffuse crackles in the chest and monocytosis.

He was a new patient for me, although the family was well known. Here was a hard-line case who despised doctors because 'they nearly killed him in hospital some years ago when he had double pneumonia'. He was neither hostile nor enthusiastic—just terribly ill and resigned to the coercion of his family.

On examination he was pale and in a cold sweat, with a feeble but regular pulse, and rattles all over the chest (back and front). He and his family hammered the previous history of double pneumonia and, to my eternal discredit, I let them divert my proper thinking. His blood count showed a monocytosis of 12 per cent = 972 absolute. Hypnotised by the pneumonia story, I thought of endocarditis complications and gave him amoxycillin. He refused to go to hospital and went home.

Next day he returned, even worse but still refusing to go to hospital. At the risk of overservicing, I did another blood count. The monocytosis had risen to 16 per cent = 1072 absolute. By now, after a good night's rest, I had shed the shackles of the double pneumonia and was back to normal thinking.

Pallor + cold sweats + shivering + monocytosis + Papua New Guinea = malaria?

Monocytosis is the only consistent abnormality in the malarial blood picture. Long ago, before Field's stain, monocytosis plus the classical symptoms in the slide-negative case were considered diagnostic. I did Field and thin films: both negative.

Old timers also taught that if large lymphocytes are well in excess of small ones in slide-negative cases, with a long past history and suggestive symptoms, the patient most probably is malarial. The ratio here, large to small, was 22 to 15. Jackpot.

As this author suffers from precisely these same rigors and so on, even 11 years after emigrating from the endemic area, the lucky patient was supplied with combined sulphadoxine and pyrimethamine plus quinine bihydrochloride from personal stock. He trotted in the next day, asymptomatic and doctor-oriented.

DISCUSSION AND LESSONS LEARNED

- This blood film method of diagnosis for malaria was a trick of the trade in the past when other investigatory methods were not available. Malaria is typically diagnosed by experienced practitioners finding parasites in erythrocytes on microscopic examination of thick and thin blood smears enhanced with Wright or Giemsa stains. Rapid diagnostic tests at the point of care have an important place. PCR and species-specific DNA probes can be used but have a limited place.

- Malaria is the super mimic. The parasites travel everywhere, and the organs in which they sporulate modify the picture to imitate any known disease.

- The classic attack is but one facet of the many-splendored *Plasmodium*. Similarly, when there are signs and symptoms that make no sense, it is odds-on positive to be malaria if there is monocytosis and the remotest connection with malaria.

- *P. falciparum* is self-limiting: *P. vivax,* like old soldiers, fades away . . . slowly. Old veterans, take heart.

Alive, well and not to be forgotten

Before World War II, Britain was dotted with infectious disease hospitals—dubbed 'fever hospitals'. Scarlet fever, diphtheria, rheumatic fever, chicken pox, whooping cough and measles were rife and often fatal. After the end of the war in 1945, the incidence and severity of the infectious diseases declined dramatically. This was due to the introduction of immunisation programs, a fall in the virulence of the streptococcus, improvement of living standards and the discovery of antibiotics. At the same time, the incidence of tuberculosis (TB) increased. Consequently, the emptying infectious disease hospitals became TB hospitals, with wards full of seriously affected children, adolescents and adults. Along came triple therapy—streptomycin, para-amino salicylic acid (PAS) and isoniazid—and the tubercle bacillus was conquered. Hospitals once more began to empty. A similar pattern occurred in Australia: tubercle was dead, or at least thought to be no longer a problem.

The Case of Mr HB

Now in his mid-70s, always dapper and very correct, Mr HB had spent the last third of the year suffering from severe sciatica with all its associated pain, analgesics and detailed investigation. Two weeks before Christmas he presented with a unilateral headache. Always a migraine sufferer, he assumed this was one of his usual attacks brought on by the persistent sciatic stress that had disallowed him the normal relaxations in his beloved garden. The story, however, did not quite ring the vasospastic bell and, sure enough, one week later the telltale blebs of herpes zoster of the ophthalmic branch of the right trigeminal nerve began to appear. As he seemed otherwise well, I had no hesitation in prescribing corticosteroids. The nasociliary branch, and therefore the eye itself, remained unaffected, and so we soldiered on through the various stages of the eruption and its attendant pain.

In March, the sciatica began to get really bad again and Mr HB also complained of a persistent dry cough. He remained well. Within the next two months he was assessed by the orthopaedic specialist, and spinal stenosis with the possibility of laminectomy was discussed. The cough had persisted. Despite the absence of clinical signs, I felt it wise to have his chest X-rayed. The report read:

> There is some patchy nodular shadowing peripherally in the
> right upper zone. There is some further nodular shadowing
> in the right lung apex. These shadows may be either recent
> or of long-standing nature.

There had been no weight loss, no night sweats, no shortness of breath and no loss of energy.

'I never told you that I was turned down for military service in 1939,' said Mr HB. 'They said I had signs of TB. I was most upset. I had never had any trouble before and have had none since.'

I referred him to our thoracic physician who phoned me later. 'When I bronchoscoped him, his bronchus was full of caseous-looking material, almost completely blocked at the right bronchus.' Mr HB was admitted to hospital. Infection with the tubercle bacillus was confirmed, and his family went through the usual surveillance. Triple therapy 'nouveau' was commenced, and Mr HB was doing very nicely after only seven days.

DISCUSSION AND LESSONS LEARNED

- Should we always order a chest X-ray of every one of our elderly patients who present with herpes zoster ophthalmicus before prescribing corticosteroids? I think not.
- Always get the patient's full story. This will guide us towards the correct path of diagnosis and management and help us avoid embarrassing pitfalls.
- Although now rare, the cause of the romantic consumption of Robert Louis Stevenson, Frédéric Chopin and *La Dame aux Camélias*, the tubercle bacillus, is alive and well and living in Australia.

Thoroughly analysing Milly

Milly presented as a dishevelled pensioner with vague undifferentiated chest pain for which she had consulted a variety of health professionals. Although the pain seemed mild, a thorough insight into her lifestyle revealed it was a major disability, and later led to her death.

The first encounter

I vividly remember my first consultation at the end of a busy Saturday morning with Milly, a 62-year-old Queenslander. Her diminutive figure was crowned with an unruly shock of hair and I felt she was yet another person losing interest in herself and living.

Milly's presenting complaint was a peculiar type of chest pain: her chest became stiff and sore after activity. She had suffered with it a long time, had tried a variety of medications and had consulted a number of general practitioners (GPs) without success.

Despite my lack of enthusiasm I took a detailed history. The problem seemed simple, the provisional diagnosis being a musculoskeletal disorder of the chest wall with angina as the differential diagnosis. After checking her blood pressure I prescribed medication and reassured her, arranging for a consultation soon after I would have the results of blood tests. On review she claimed to be free of the pain and requested permission to participate in a lawn bowls pennant competition later in the week. Surprised, I agreed.

The merry-go-round

Milly consulted me four weeks later when she admitted the pain was so severe that she had sought the aid of a chiropractor and a physiotherapist. The pain had persisted and she consulted another doctor who referred her to an orthopaedic specialist. She was returning to my care because I had given her the most relief. At each consultation she gave the impression of a tired, depressed and lonely pensioner.

Milly presented four months later with severe chest pain. Cardiac enzyme studies were consistent with recent myocardial infarction, confirmed by electrocardiogram (ECG), which also revealed a left bundle branch block.

The home visit—the 'real' patient

Milly's small home was immaculate. It was clean and fresh inside and outside. The carefully manicured garden was a picture. Everything had the mark of a houseproud perfectionist.

I took renewed interest in her with the realisation that the tired little lady I had been seeing in the surgery was not the 'real' Milly. It became obvious that the mild chest pain was a major disabling problem. She was unable to bowl as usual, nor was she able to participate in her beloved ballroom dancing. Colleagues at her bowling club gave a new picture of Milly. She was a tireless worker, extremely active and always neat and tidy, but her friends had noticed a recent lack of interest in her appearance.

Managing her angina was difficult but possible with judicious juggling of drugs. I advised Milly that angiography with a view to coronary artery bypass surgery was appropriate. She flatly refused and expressed her greatest fear: some complication would force her to become an inpatient in a nursing home or hospital where she could not pursue full community life. I continued to manage Milly conservatively.

Milly resumed ballroom dancing, albeit with less vigour, and won the State Singles Lawn Bowls Championship for the second time in three years, giving her a feeling of joy and self-worth.

The final home visit

One month after the bowling triumph I was called to her home after the Saturday evening dance. She had classic symptoms of angina, rapidly relieved by standard medication. She settled and rested.

Milly's neighbour rang early Sunday morning and I sensed something was seriously wrong with Milly. At her home I found her dead in bed; she had apparently died quietly and peacefully in her sleep.

DISCUSSION AND LESSONS LEARNED

- The significance of chest pain is highlighted yet again. Coronary artery disease is the primary differential diagnosis of every patient with unusual chest pain, which should be regarded as coronary in origin until proved otherwise.
- The disability of patients who may be stoic in nature or who may have personality problems should be recognised and respected.
- Milly epitomises an important learning experience for general practitioners. Home visits allow a first-hand knowledge of the way patients behave in their own environment and this helps us to know them as people. Impressions from surgery consultations often are half-impressions. Unless doctors make appropriate house calls to determine where, how and why people live as they do, they will never know their patients adequately.
- Milly's case also highlights the right of competent adult patients to refuse recommended treatment. We often think of consent as when the patient agrees to our recommended investigations and treatment but an adult patient who has capacity can refuse any intervention, even if this results in death.

A pain in the butt

John R, a 50-year-old accountant, was an avid ballroom dancer and tennis player, but his activity was curtailed by persistent low-back pain and right-leg pain. Pain in his back and right buttock would radiate into his thigh and calf after only five minutes of dancing or tennis.

He was referred to me for an epidural injection to alleviate his back pain and sciatica. An accompanying X-ray confirmed degeneration of his L5–S1 intervertebral disc. Examination of his lumbosacral spine revealed tenderness at this level and restricted flexion and extension movements. At follow-up four weeks later, he claimed that the injection had not helped.

Diagnosis and outcome

The penny dropped when I reflected on the nature of the pain. Despite his relative youth he obviously had vascular claudication. He was a moderate smoker. In addition, he claimed his erections were 'not as good as they should be'.

Following exercise, auscultation revealed a loud bruit over the aortic bifurcation, the right common iliac artery and the right femoral artery. The peripheral pulses were weaker in his right leg. I referred him to a vascular surgeon who ordered an angiogram (Figure 2.1), which confirmed arterial disease, including a tight stenosis in his right common iliac artery and the left internal iliac with an aneurysm in the distal part of the left common iliac artery. John underwent aorto bi-iliac Dacron grafting (Figure 2.2) and for the past 18 years has been untroubled by leg pain, although he has suffered a myocardial infarction.

DISCUSSION AND LESSONS LEARNED

- When an older patient presents with the common problem of 'sciatica', the possibility of peripheral vascular (arterial) disease (PVD) must be considered.
- If the patient has PVD, risk factors including smoking, hypercholesterolaemia, hypertension and diabetes mellitus must be considered, as should precipitating factors such as beta-blocker therapy and anaemia.

- There is invariably an associated risk with generalised atherosclerosis and I have encountered many patients who have suffered myocardial infarction or a stroke during or after surgery.
- With an increasing ageing population we are seeing a concomitant rise in problems of claudication, both vascular and neurogenic (due to spinal canal stenosis). The presentation of neurogenic claudication in fact is almost identical to that of John R.

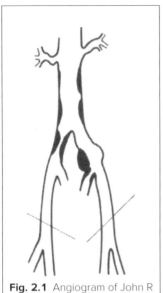

Fig. 2.1 Angiogram of John R

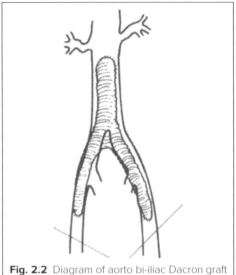

Fig. 2.2 Diagram of aorto bi-iliac Dacron graft of John R

Polymyalgia rheumatica: mimic supreme

Mrs Gulliver

Mrs Gulliver, a widow who had just had her 50th birthday, was always smartly dressed and neatly coiffured, and she presented well. Fay, her only child, was 13 years old. Mrs Gulliver sat straight before me, head forward, shiny eyes staring straight into mine. 'You must tell me the absolute truth, Doctor.'

The absolute truth in the report on my desk was most unkind: 'The mediastinum is enlarged and there is presence of a mass in the superior and anterior mediastinum . . . I would consider in particular bronchogenic neoplasm.' I thought of her 30 cigarettes a day for 20 years. I also thought of the small supraclavicular lymph nodes seen by one of my partners about a year ago and the dysphagia (barium swallow negative) complained of six months before.

Mrs Gulliver had presented two months ago complaining of morning stiffness and pain affecting neck, trapezius and deltoid muscles. She was extremely tender and the pain made her miserable. She had had a previous rotator cuff problem. 'This is different,' she declared. Erythrocyte sedimentation rate (ESR) was 65, white cell count (WCC) 12 000, and my heart leapt at the magic response to prednisone. But every time I tried to reduce the dose, the pain and stiffness recurred. She latterly complained of a persistent cough and full feeling in the middle of the chest; thus the disastrous chest X-ray.

Mr Fredericks

Mr Fredericks, an 80-year-old, had developed during his past 10 years a potpourri of pathology tic douloureux, atrial fibrillation with congestive cardiac failure, severe diverticular disease, and the expected degenerative disease of cervical spine and shoulder joints. His main complaint became severe pain affecting neck and shoulder girdle and hips, worse in the night and early morning, with associated stiffness. He did not respond to physiotherapy or anti-inflammatory medication. A full blood examination showed an ESR of 57. A presumptive diagnosis of polymyalgia rheumatica was made and a therapeutic trial of prednisone commenced. The improvement was definite and dramatic and allowed him to return to his physical work on a somewhat large piece of land. This improvement continued, if less positively, over a period of six months until he asked for a home visit because of the severe intractable pain affecting neck, shoulders and upper back.

He was referred for an opinion:

> Just a follow-up note on this gentleman whom I admitted to hospital on 13 October. At that time I noticed that he had been treated for polymyalgia since July 1986 with prednisone. Over the preceding 3 weeks he had developed severe upper thoracic

pain, which had made him bedridden. There had been some associated night sweats and he had severe tenderness over thoracic vertebrae four. This was associated with a fever of 37.5 °C. He had irritability of his hips and shoulders. Clinically he appeared to have a crush fracture of T4 and this was confirmed on X-ray. Rectal examination showed an extremely hard prostate. A bone scan showed multiple foci of increased uptake in the thora-columbar spine, sacrum, both shoulders, ribs, pelvis and both proximal femora. A prostatic biopsy was performed and this confirmed adenocarcinoma.

It would appear unlikely that he does have true polymyalgia rheumatica.

Orchidectomy and radiotherapy induced pain relief and for some months at least he was able to return to normal activities. How the mighty are fallen.

DISCUSSION AND LESSONS LEARNED

- Polymyalgia rheumatica can be a snare and a delusion. Commonly underdiagnosed and undertreated, unfortunately it may also be misdiagnosed and mistreated. The danger for a general practitioner is that, having seen a few proven and successfully relieved cases, there may be a tendency to be over-smart and under-careful in the approach to new presentations. Malignancy must always be excluded.
- The rules remain the same—listen to the patient and examine carefully all aspects before embarking on a program of treatment. General practice is not easy.

Coeliac disease: a disease of many faces and ages

Jack, aged 15 months, was brought by his parents because of increasing diarrhoea with six large offensive stools daily. He had been seen by another doctor four weeks earlier who considered an infective cause but stool microscopy and culture showed no parasites and no growth of pathogens. A trial of tinidazole seemed to aggravate the diarrhoea. He was unwell, anorexic, miserable and irritable, had abdominal bloating and had lost weight. Jack seemed to thrive when breast fed for 10 months and only started eating solid food four months ago. He was diagnosed as having coeliac disease.

Siobhan, aged 32 years, presented with several days of malaise, lethargy and mouth ulcers. Over the past 10 months she had suffered from flatulence and bloating in addition to loose bowel actions about three times a day interspersed with short periods of constipation. She described ongoing fatigue and weight loss of 8 kg over this time. On examination she was a pale, thin, tall woman with no subcutaneous fat. Diagnosis: coeliac disease.

Cathy, aged 46, gave this testimony to our local newspaper: 'My coeliac disease was picked up by accident as I was asymptomatic. It started two years before that when my teenage daughter was quite sick, always complaining of tummy pains and being tired. We went to seven specialists in 18 months. They looked at everything and finally tested for coeliac disease. Her blood tests were sky-high so the family had to be tested and I came back positive. I had a biopsy which gave the positive diagnosis. Being diagnosed has been the best thing as we've got a totally new lease on life'.

DISCUSSION AND LESSONS LEARNED

- The above three case histories highlight the variable presentations of coeliac disease which has the classic tetrad of diarrhoea, weight loss, iron/folate deficiency and abdominal bloating.
- Children usually develop it between 9 and 18 months of age following the introduction of solids into the diet. They usually present as failure to thrive.
- Coeliac disease may affect people of all ages, and it is just as likely to be recognised in those over 60 years of age as it is in infancy and the first two decades of life.
- The serological diagnostic screening tests are total IgA level and IgA transglutaminase antibodies. If these are positive irrespective of titre, refer for the gold standard test of small bowel biopsy, which may reveal the characteristic villous atrophy.

Chest pain of unusual cause

Roger G, aged 66, was a retired retail manager who presented with several days of dull pleuritic chest pain radiating to the left side of the chest.

He had a history of a myocardial infarction 20 years previously and recent transient ischaemia attacks for which he had been prescribed warfarin. This treatment was suspended following a bleeding duodenal ulcer. He responded well to triple therapy. He also suffered from diabetes and glaucoma.

Examination revealed evidence only of chronic obstructive airway disease. This clinical diagnosis was confirmed on a chest X-ray, which also showed a slightly enlarged heart shadow and an unfolding of the aorta. Other tests included cardiac enzymes, which were normal, and a full blood count, which showed Hb 11.0 g/dL, WCC 4100, platelets 187 000, Na 137 mmol/L, K 4.0 mmol/L, Cl 81 mmol/L, Ca 2.35 mmol/L. Urinalysis was clear.

An ECG showed an old inferior infarction and normal sinus rhythm but no recent changes. A diagnosis of 'chest wall syndrome' was made and the patient was given supportive and symptomatic treatment. However, because the chest pain persisted, and as an infolding of the thoracic aorta was reported on chest X-ray, a CT (computerised tomography) scan of the thorax was ordered and it was reported as normal.

Roger was referred to a physician who repeated the chest X-ray. This X-ray showed a crush fracture as well as moderate osteoporosis in the vertebrae.

Diagnosis and outcome

Roger was admitted to hospital for a series of tests. These included a bone marrow cytological aspirate and a bone scan. The bone marrow biopsy showed plasmacytosis with atypical primitive and multinucleated forms. The bone scan showed multiple malignant deposits in the ribs and in the skull. In particular, there was increased uptake in the left first rib and absent foci of uptake in the inferior pole of the sternum.

A further CT scan showed changes of myeloma: multiple lytic areas with wedging at T8 and compression of the body of L5 and some destruction of L4.

The diagnosis now was non-secretory multiple myeloma. The chest pain was secondary to myeloma lesions in the thoracic vertebrae.

Roger was treated with regular courses of melphalan and prednisone, plus lenalidomide. His complete blood count was monitored and he received analgesics when required. He died three years after presentation.

DISCUSSION AND LESSONS LEARNED

- Multiple myeloma can certainly be a difficult disease to detect in its early stages as it is developing in bone. It may simply present as mild regional pain, especially of the back.
- One of the best ways to detect it is by an abnormally high ESR, which unfortunately was not performed as an initial screening procedure. Anaemia is also a feature, and in retrospect the haemoglobin of 11.0 g/dL was an early pointer that was overlooked.
- It can also present as mild osteoporosis on plain X-ray in its early stages, but significant radiological changes may not declare until the disease is well advanced. The importance of a bone scan if malignancy is suspected is highlighted in this patient.

An unusual presentation of a common disorder

Day 1—Tuesday

Miss M W, aged 8, presented with epigastric pains. There were no other symptoms.

She had a low-grade fever, the right iliac fossa was mildly tender and bowel sounds were slightly hyperactive. However, she appeared quite well and had no significant past history.

A tentative diagnosis of early appendicitis or viral mesenteric adenitis was made. There was no reason to consider functional disease high among the diagnostic probabilities. She was discharged to her mother's care for observation at home and general advice on follow-up was given.

Day 4—Friday morning

M's pain had been smouldering but there were no new symptoms. She appeared to be generally well and was quite cheerful. The low-grade fever continued: she now had mild tenderness in the right upper quadrant but the liver was impalpable and there was no jaundice. No urine specimen was available for testing; no other physical abnormalities were detected despite an exhaustive examination.

Hepatitis was promoted now to the head of the list of diagnostic probabilities despite a negative history of contact. The mother was asked to check the colour of urine and faeces and was given general advice. No pharmacological action was taken nor had proprietary analgesics been given.

The mother later phoned to say that M's urine was dark. She was asked to bring in a urine specimen.

Day 4—Friday afternoon

M's urine was indeed dark and testing was positive—not for bilirubin but for blood; there was no proteinuria. With a working diagnosis of glomerulonephritis, a most searching history was unhelpful and a repeated physical examination still revealed only mild tenderness in the right upper quadrant. She was asked to return with an early morning specimen.

Day 5—Saturday morning

M returned with a urine specimen that was still positive (+ +) for blood but otherwise was normal. An additional symptom now had appeared: her bowel motions that morning were black and tarry. An occult blood test was positive.

The working diagnosis now centred on haemorrhagic diatheses such as Henoch–Schönlein or idiopathic thrombocytopenic purpura. However, there was no splenomegaly, no lymphadenopathy, no clinical jaundice, no masses, no rash and no other clinical evidence of haemorrhagic disorder such as bruising or petechiae; heart sounds were dual.

Day 5—Saturday afternoon

An urgent full blood examination, ESR and clotting profile gave a diagnosis. The clotting parameters were marginally impaired, ESR was 10, and the red cell parameters were normal and the white cell count was within normal limits; but a differential count revealed 50 per cent atypical lymphocytes, and serology confirmed a diagnosis of glandular fever. Urine microscopy had confirmed the dipstick finding of haematuria. Even with a diagnosis firmly established, no clinical evidence of Epstein–Barr mononucleosis could be found.

On the assumption that her haematuria and melaena reflected impaired hepatic function, M was given 10 mg of vitamin K by intramuscular injection.

Day 6—Sunday

Urine was still weakly positive (trace) for non-haemolysed blood; bowel motions were still dark. Submandibular node enlargement was detected for the first time. The liver and spleen were impalpable and the nodes elsewhere were normal. There was no rash.

Day 8—Tuesday

The submandibular nodes were now unmistakeably enlarged. There was no fever, pharyngitis or rash. Lymph nodes elsewhere were normal. Both the liver and the spleen were enlarged but neither was tender. Urinalysis was normal and the mother reported that bowel motions were now a normal colour and consistency.

M had remained clinically well and cheerful throughout the course of her illness and was under a customary conservative management regime. Subsequently she developed the typical purplish rash of infectious (Epstein–Barr) mononucleosis on the lower abdomen.

DISCUSSION AND LESSONS LEARNED

- This case is presented not only as a diagnostic conundrum but also as an illustration of a systemic illness presenting with manifestations in many organs other than those that first come to mind when the illness is named.
- Primarily, M's case shows that when a symptom complex suggests a specific diagnosis the practitioner must take care that he or she is not blinded by his or her own (or another's) diagnostic label. He or she should

be sensitive to changes in the clinical story—which rarely will be as apparent as those described above—and should be prepared to revise the diagnosis in the light of those changes.

She was, of course, a doctor's wife

The history started on a Friday evening. The patient had been unusually quiet on the way down with her husband to their seaside cottage for the weekend and during dinner developed sudden and severe rigors. She had been perfectly well up to this time—a minor non-extractive dental procedure had been performed two to three weeks previously.

Rigors continued intermittently during the next two days. The husband, who was wont to be critical of the fact that many doctors—particularly the younger ones—no longer carried thermometers as part of their home visiting kit, just happened to have one in his pocket. He noted that, while afebrile in the evening, the temperature, coincident with a rigor, reached 41°C in the early hours of the morning.

On Monday morning the blood picture, including the ESR, was shown to be completely normal. There was no pus in the urine, and an X-ray of the chest was clear apart from calcification of the mitral valve, which an experienced radiologist pointed out was present in the ring and was not involving the cusps. There was no lymphadenopathy, no splenomegaly or liver enlargement, but a pansystolic mitral murmur, known to be present for some years, seemed rougher and louder. The husband referred the patient, fairly sure that he was about to be involved in only the second case of infective endocarditis seen in his medical lifetime.

The physician to whom the patient was referred tended to agree. She developed just palpable splenomegaly, the rigors continued daily, and apart from the cardiac bruit, no further abnormal physical signs were found. Or rather the husband-doctor did not think so. A capable registrar thought he could hear a mitral diastolic murmur as well as one at the left sternal border, and a cardiologist who came with his echocardiograph demonstrated what he maintained were vegetations on both valves.

The husband, who had been brought up on mere stethoscope diagnosis of valve lesions, was somewhat unconvinced and uncharitably suggested that perhaps some of the green flashes could have been due to a loose wire or something in the machine he had never been quite so close to before. Nevertheless, in spite of repeatedly negative blood cultures—a dozen or so in the first five days—he was importunate enough to press the physician captain of the team to do something, even to the extent of starting intravenous penicillin, although this would mean long-term commitment.

In the meantime, blood pictures remained normal, unlikely parasites had been looked for, exotic agglutinations done, and chest X-rays and ECGs remained unchanged.

On the morning of the seventh day the mononuclear cells in the film were declared atypical and foamy, the Paul–Bunnell became positive to a titre of 1/1280, and the rigors ceased. No prodromal illness, no sore throat or pharyngeal exudate, no lymphadenopathy, minimal splenomegaly?

She was, of course, a doctor's wife.

The sinister modern pestilence

Adam R, a 23-year-old laboratory technician, presented with a one-week history of a sore throat, headache, fever and lethargy. Examination revealed a temperature of 38.1 °C, pharyngitis and cervical lymphadenopathy. I ordered a Paul–Bunnell test and took a throat swab, which produced negative results. I then instructed him to take the penicillin I had prescribed.

He returned in five days saying that he felt worse, and he had now developed a rash. The rash was a fine salmon-pink maculopapular rash on the upper trunk and extremities, and it included the palms of the hand. This made me wonder about secondary syphilis, but I thought it more likely to be a viral exanthema or a drug reaction. In addition, enlarged nodes were now palpable in the groin and he had hepatomegaly. I thought that it must be Epstein–Barr mononucleosis and ordered more blood tests.

On review he had developed a painful rash on his face: herpes zoster affecting the ophthalmic division of the 5th cranial nerve.

Diagnosis and outcome

It was time to consider human immunodeficiency virus (HIV) infection and so I ordered HIV screening tests; these were positive. The process of breaking the news to Adam was the really difficult step. He was referred to a specialist clinic and died two years later.

DISCUSSION AND LESSONS LEARNED

- HIV infection seems to be here to stay, and as primary-care physicians we have to be watchful for the early symptoms and signs of the infection. Without a high degree of suspicion, the diagnosis can frequently be missed. Like diseases such as infectious mononucleosis, diabetes mellitus and malignancy, HIV infection can develop surreptitiously and be difficult to diagnose in its early stages.

- Early clinical features include unexplained fever, sore throat, malaise, diarrhoea, chronic cough and headache. About 75 per cent of patients develop an acute mononucleosis-like illness about two to four weeks after infection with HIV. There are very many skin signs of HIV infection. Apart from Kaposi's sarcoma and the typical fine maculopapular rash, HIV infection should be suspected in young persons with shingles and atypical herpes simplex.

- These patients need our personal support and understanding; considerable sensitivity, tact and kindness should always accompany breaking the news to patients. Fortunately, with modern antimicrobials, outcomes continue to improve 15 years following Adam's 'tale'.

Premarital syphilis or a rash decision?

Josie M, a 21-year-old university student, presented in great distress on the eve of her wedding. She had developed a coarse dark-pink rash over most of her body five days previously and was informed by the young doctor at the university health service that she probably had secondary syphilis: 'The rash is typical; I'll start you on penicillin and organise some special blood tests'. (Refer to Figure 2.3, centre insert page 1.)

Josie, who came from a very religious family was 'numb with disbelief. Here I am getting married in two days to the only man I have ever loved and I'm told I have syphilis. Can you believe it? Could I have picked it up from a toilet? Surely Peter couldn't have it—he's so faithful. Look at me, I have this unsightly rash on the neck and chest and I'm supposed to look beautiful on my wedding day'.

Diagnosis and outcome

While I was looking at the rash (as Josie wept) and fighting feelings of disbelief at such stupidity from a colleague, I inquired, 'Did you notice a roundish mark on your skin before the rash appeared all over your body?'

'Yes—around my tummy. I thought it must have been a ringworm I picked up on the farm.' Yes, Josie had the common problem of pityriasis rosea. Josie went off happily with appropriate reassurance, advice about make up for the rash on exposed parts and some undeserved support for my colleague ('This rash tricks us all the time—I had never heard about it in my medical course but I heard a lot about syphilis'). Josie lived happily ever after (well, for about seven years until she was divorced).

DISCUSSION AND LESSONS LEARNED

- Never make diagnoses, especially on sensitive and emotional problems, unless absolutely sure.
- Skin rashes are vast in number and type and are even baffling for dermatologists; we should refer if in doubt. The tendency also to diagnose any rash as dermatitis and prescribe corticosteroids is unacceptable practice.
- Pityriasis rosea is a common rash with a variable distribution. We need to be watchful lest we misdiagnose it.

All that wheezes is not asthma

Case 1

The story of Sue W, an international university student, was brought to my attention when I was asked to prepare a report for a medical defence organisation. She presented to the university student health service with three months of coughing, wheezing and dyspnoea on exertion. The problem was diagnosed as bronchial asthma and salbutamol was prescribed. The patient reported back in one week and said that she felt only slightly improved, so a combined corticosteroid and beta-agonist inhaler was prescribed. She reported a significant improvement at first but then said she developed a cold with a persistent fever and the respiratory symptoms were worse. She was then prescribed a short course of oral corticosteroids.

Eventually Sue was discovered comatose by her flatmate. She was taken to hospital, where she was found to have miliary tuberculosis and tuberculoid meningitis. According to her flatmate she gradually deteriorated with weight loss and weakness, became frustrated, confused and irritable, and refused to seek medical attention. She still remains in a semi-coma in her home country and requires constant nursing care. The medico-legal consequences were massive.

Case 2

Another medico-legal case was that of a 25-year-old white, South African woman who was visiting Australia on an extended holiday to see relatives. She visited a country practice complaining of coughing and wheezing. She was also treated for bronchial asthma for several weeks before pulmonary tuberculosis was diagnosed on chest X-ray.

Case 3

The Melbourne *Herald Sun* of 27 March 2017 reported:

> *A deadly outbreak of drug resistant tuberculosis has occurred in Australia because a Sydney doctor wrongly diagnosed a 23-year-old university student with asthma and then lung cancer before realising it was TB.*
>
> *A further 10 people were infected by the disease after the man tried to get treatment from his GP and only after his third return visit—and three months of sickness—was referred for an X-ray which uncovered a 6 cm hole in his lung. Patient zero was informed that his persistent cough, shortness of breath and general malaise was likely lung cancer. Hospital*

investigation confirmed that he was suffering from a slightly drug-resistant strain of tuberculosis.

DISCUSSION AND LESSONS LEARNED

- All that wheezes is not asthma and certainly not in visitors, migrants and refugees from other countries, particularly Africa and the Asian sub-continent. Tuberculosis is now a common finding in refugees. Children are especially vulnerable.
- The importance of a routine chest X-ray early after presentation becomes obvious.
- Tuberculosis is diagnosed by a Mantoux test, sputum or gastric aspirate for gram stain and culture, and interferon gamma release assay (IGRA). The new immunochromatographic finger-prick test is a promising test.
- Always consider HIV in a patient with TB.
- Special care is needed to avoid corticosteroid use in patients suspected of harbouring tuberculosis.

Great mimics: some concluding reflections

The great mimics of the past were the notorious infections: syphilis and tuberculosis. A host of other infections and neurological disorders also represented past mimics. The major diseases of modern Western society, atherosclerosis and malignant disease, have replaced the great infections of the past century as the major life-threatening diseases. Surprisingly, atherosclerosis in its various manifestations of coronary artery disease, cerebrovascular disease and peripheral vascular disease can mimic a number of conditions and the diagnosis can be difficult initially. Malignant disease, especially lymphoma, multiple myeloma and carcinoma of the central nervous system, lungs, kidney, caecum and other internal organs or 'silent areas', can mimic a variety of diseases.

The infections, malaria and Epstein–Barr mononucleosis, as represented in this chapter are mimics, and we must not forget HIV, tuberculosis and syphilis. Other important mimics include the various endocrine disorders and the rheumatic or connective tissue diseases such as systemic lupus erythematosus, polymyositis and polymyalgia rheumatica.

Masquerades and pitfalls

Chapter 3

Four brief histories of a 'great pretender'

Case 1

A 32-year-old woman presented with 12 months of fluctuating symptoms of polyarthritis of the proximal (PIP) and distal interphalangeal joints (DIP) of the hand. Other symptoms included malaise, fever, mouth ulceration and Raynaud's phenomenon. The only abnormal findings were evidence of Raynaud's phenomenon in fingers, palmar erythema and mild fever but no deformity of the joints of the hand.

Case 2

A 56-year-old farmer presented with three months of painful, swollen hands, wrists, feet and knees. Associated symptoms included severe fatigue, morning stiffness, intermittent grittiness of the eyes and dryness of the mouth. On examination he had synovial thickening and tenderness in the metacarpophalangeal (MCP) and PIP joints and the knees. He also had a dry mouth and conjunctivitis of the left eye.

Case 3

A 17-year-old female student presented with 10 weeks of pain in her hands, wrists, knees, ankles, feet and shoulders. She also had swelling of the ankles and morning stiffness. She had been taking minocycline for acne for 12 months. Examination revealed tenderness of the left third PIP joint only.

Case 4

A 30-year-old salesman presented with 10 days of shortness of breath, cough, night sweats and chest pain. He described 12 months of mild, variable, intermittent pain of his hands, wrists and shoulders. On examination he had mild synovitis of the MCP and PIP joints of both hands and bilateral pleural effusions.

DISCUSSION AND LESSONS LEARNED

These four patients all had systemic lupus erythematosus (SLE) which is a multisystemic autoimmune connective tissue disorder with a multitude of clinical symptoms and a wide variety of presentations (Hanrahan, 2001). These include dermatological, neurological, cardiovascular, haematological, renal and obstetric manifestations. However, the two most common symptoms are joint pain and fatigue. SLE is associated with multiple drug allergies as exemplified in Case 3 (tetracyclines) and should be considered in young females with problems with the oral contraceptive pill and pregnancy. For suspected SLE the recommended approach is to perform an antinuclear (ANA) test and, if positive, order dsDNA and ENA antibodies—especially Sm.

The dramatic tale of 'Hollywood Tom'— surgeon extraordinaire

Tom was a popular medical colleague who was the envy of many because of his debonair bronze surfie looks and immaculate presentation. In fact he was so suave and attractive to the ladies that we called him 'Hollywood Tom'. He reminded me of Charles Dickens' Dr Jobling who was described thus:

> *His neckerchief and shirt frill were ever of the whitest; his*
> *clothes were of the blackest and slickest, his gold watch-*
> *chain of the heaviest and his seals of the largest. His boots,*
> *which were of the brightest, creaked as he walked—and he*
> *had a peculiar way of smacking his lips and saying 'ah'*

at intervals while patients detailed their symptoms, which inspired great confidence.

(Charles Dickens, *The Life and Adventures of Martin Chuzzlewit,* 1844s)

Over the years, Tom always looked a picture of health, with his hallmark swarthy looks. He did not smoke and only drank alcohol socially.

At a medical reunion we observed that the 60-year-old surgeon looked tired and thin. He confided that he was very tired and concerned about his weight loss. He did not have a general practitioner and had not sought a consultation but said that he was coming to see me for a check up. However, in a few days time we heard the sad news that his left leg suddenly gave way and he collapsed to the floor. He had a pathological fracture of the femur due to a metastatic deposit from a hepatoma, which had developed in a cirrhotic liver caused by primary haemochromatosis. Tom died about five months later.

DISCUSSION AND LESSONS LEARNED

- Osler's aphorism comes to mind: 'The doctor who treats himself has a fool for a patient'.
- All doctors should have their own general practitioner and ideally present for regular consultation especially in areas of prevention. Indeed, 'Good medical practice: a code of conduct for doctors in Australia' states that good medical practice involves:
  - having a general practitioner
  - seeking independent, objective advice when you need medical care, and being aware of the risks of self-diagnosis and self-treatment.
- If we notice any unusual pigmentation we should think of the relatively common condition of haemochromatosis and also Addison's disease and an adverse drug effect. Tom's continuing and deepening 'tan' was obviously the progression of his disorder.

- We keep being surprised by the frequency of the diagnosis of haemochromatosis in our patient population even in the very elderly and we should be more mindful of it. It is worth asking about a family history in our routine medical history of a new patient.

Getting out of rhythm

Two cases

'Will you come and see Uncle Sam please—he's having another of his mini strokes.' Stroke number nine in fact! It was my very first week in country practice and I was bemused by the call. Sam P, a 72-year-old farmer, was quite well apart from his blackouts and, like doctors before me, I could find absolutely nothing wrong with him. Apparently he would suddenly black out and recover after a few minutes. I asked him to arrange a consultation the following day.

Evelyn A, aged 68, was another local identity who complained *ad nauseam* about vague feelings of fatigue, lack of energy and occasional light headedness. After several visits to various doctors (including specialists) she would dismiss it as 'getting old—but I hate not being my usual fit self'.

Diagnoses and outcomes

Both Sam and Evelyn had the problem of bradyarrhythmia—a paroxysmal cardiac abnormality that can be very difficult to detect. Sam's complete heart block disorder, manifesting as Stokes–Adams attacks, was diagnosed by admitting him to hospital and attaching our brand new cardiac monitor (this was 1970).

Evelyn's sick sinus syndrome was diagnosed using a 24-hour Holter ambulatory ECG. It was disturbing to realise that she had suffered with its manifestations for six years before the cause of her sluggishness and light headedness was determined.

The two patients were given a new lease of life with the insertion of pacemakers. Sam (Refer to Figure 3.1, centre insert page 1) was given one of the first pacemakers in our part of the country.

DISCUSSION AND LESSONS LEARNED

- Cardiac arrhythmias should be considered in any person presenting with dizziness, blackouts or uncharacteristic poor health, including lethargy and exertional dyspnoea. Pacing should be considered in these circumstances and also with incipient cardiac failure or angina. It can be a most insidious problem and a difficult one to diagnose, as well as being fatal. The use of a 24-hour Holter monitor is an excellent investigatory method.
- I have never forgotten the case of a 42-year-old woman who had complete heart block and was found alive by an attendant in the cool room of a Melbourne mortuary. She had been pronounced dead at the emergency centre of one of our hospitals.
- Sometimes we tend to stop thinking and investigating when colleagues, especially those whom we consider far superior and wiser, have not been able to solve a patient's problem. Experience has taught me that one person's perception is as good as the next and that a fresh look can lead to a fresh solution.

Paling into significance

My relative, Joy T, aged 65, initially 'consulted' me at a family gathering. She described a problem of extreme fatigue: 'I cannot get out of my own way—I feel so weak'. The fatigue, which had been getting progressively worse over the past four months or so, was associated with weakness, anorexia and 'depression'. Furthermore, she complained of dyspnoea and chest tightness on moderate exertion, with occasional palpitations.

She had a history of a myocardial infarction three years before with subsequent congestive cardiac failure. She also had a 12-year history of late-onset bronchial asthma requiring maintenance oral prednisolone of 5 to 10 mg. Her medication was digoxin 0.125 mg, amiloride 5 mg–hydrochlorothiazide 50 mg (Moduretic), beclomethasone and salbutamol nebulisers, and prednisolone 10 mg daily.

She certainly looked unwell and so I advised her to return to her general practitioner as soon as possible for review. After examining her, he mentioned that her 'chest was in poor shape and that the heart was faster than normal'.

Joy's general practitioner referred her to her cardiologist who performed a battery of tests including an electrocardiogram, chest X-ray and serum electrolytes. He informed her that unfortunately she had deteriorating cardiac failure and that her potassium was too low. He prescribed potassium supplements and increased her digoxin to 0.25 mg.

Four weeks later Joy contacted me to say that she felt no better, was very depressed, had lost weight and wished that she could die.

Diagnostic probabilities

When contemplating her problem on my way to see her, I thought that she could have digitalis toxicity and perhaps diabetes mellitus (especially being on a thiazide diuretic and prednisolone); alternatively, she could have a psychological problem such as depression. However, when I saw her the striking feature was her pallor. 'Everyone says I'm grey but the specialist said it was due to my heart,' she said. I decided to order a full blood examination, serum digoxin and random blood sugar.

I was not surprised when the results revealed a haemoglobin of 67 g /L, due to iron deficiency. She had no history of bleeding but a faecal occult blood test was positive.

Diagnosis and outcome

Joy was admitted to hospital for blood transfusion and endoscopy. Gastroscopy revealed severe oesophagitis at its lower end. The conclusion was that her iron deficiency anaemia resulted from oesophagitis, possibly caused by corticosteroid therapy.

DISCUSSION AND LESSONS LEARNED

- This was an extraordinary case of a serious problem being overlooked by practitioners who appeared to have 'blinkers on' and could not think beyond the pre-existing cardiac problem. This is a modern phenomenon, and some specialists appear to have tunnel vision. As general practitioners (family physicians), we regret the apparent demise of the good general physician. The challenge is for us to adopt that generalist role and manage it competently.

- The diagnosis of anaemia should be considered in people with a history of arteriosclerosis who develop deterioration of symptoms, including angina pectoris, congestive cardiac failure (especially exertional dyspnoea) and intermittent claudication.
- Dealing with the problems of relatives can be extremely difficult, especially intervening on their behalf and potentially running into conflict with colleagues. It raises the important issue of the substandard care some patients receive if they do not have a caring competent practitioner to take responsibility for their welfare. Although whenever possible we should avoid providing medical care to anyone with whom we have a close personal relationship, we can still act as advocates for our relatives and help them to navigate the healthcare system.

The high-spirited schoolteacher

Mrs EP, a 55-year-old divorced schoolteacher, first presented to me complaining of a two-week history of proximal muscle pain and weakness in her shoulders and, to a lesser extent, her pelvic muscles. She was tired and lethargic.

My eyes lit up as I confidently made a provisional diagnosis of polymyalgia rheumatica—classic textbook material.

Initial management

An ESR of 51 supported my provisional diagnosis and so I commenced her on 30 mg prednisolone. She returned earlier than the arranged weekly review complaining of worsening symptoms. Because she lived alone, with little support, I decided to admit her under my care to the local hospital. She eagerly agreed to this decision. The plan in hospital was to continue with the steroids, provide an opportunity for rest and await the expected improvement.

A negative response

However, the plan changed as she continued to complain of muscle pain and tenderness despite continued corticosteroids. I became uneasy about the diagnosis of polymyalgia rheumatica. I arranged investigations to exclude other inflammatory and connective tissue disorders and sought an opinion from a rheumatologist. On his advice, in the presence of a rising ESR (now 79), the provisional diagnosis remained unchanged. However, the dose of steroid was increased to 50 mg daily.

General confusion

After a few days in hospital, Mrs EP became confused and complained of severe lower abdominal pains associated with nausea and frequent non-watery bowel motions. She also complained of electrical feelings through her body and other hallucinations. Examination revealed marked lower abdominal tenderness but no signs of peritonitis. Concerned about the possibility of an acute bowel perforation (secondary to the high steroid dosage), I asked a surgeon to assess her (despite normal plain abdominal X-rays). His diagnosis of acute diverticulitis (aggravated by the steroids) was confirmed by a barium enema. She settled well on intravenous antibiotics and analgesia. At the same time serum electrolytes, a full blood count and liver function tests were performed. To my surprise her liver function tests were abnormal, with marked elevation of gamma glutamyl transferase and alkaline phosphatase, consistent with alcoholic liver disease. This was a salutary lesson to me, as up to that point I had never inquired specifically about her alcohol intake, nor had it entered my mind to do so in the clinical context.

In retrospect, Mrs EP's odd behaviour soon after admission was probably an acute brain syndrome (due to alcohol withdrawal) rather than related to her medications or underlying illness.

Management and counselling

I felt it was important to confront her with these results and ascertain an exact indication of her level of alcohol consumption. After a brief period of denial, she admitted to consuming increasingly larger quantities of alcohol—in the order of one flagon of sherry daily.

For the next few days the focus of my daily visits changed from concentrating on the biological disease to helping her cope with her drinking problem. With the strengthening of the doctor–patient relationship her ability to discuss personal problems increased. It became evident that she had a full complement of risk factors, which had been previously overlooked.

A consultant (with a special interest in alcohol abuse) visited her in hospital and she developed a good working relationship with him. Various members of the hospital's nursing staff also provided valuable support over the first few days. Mrs EP found solace in religion and received a constant stream of visitors from her church community, who were able to provide the reassurance and confidence that she needed.

After nearly three weeks in hospital, she was discharged and a good network of support arranged. After six weeks her liver function tests had returned to normal and she states that she has not had a drink since. Soon she returned to teaching and appears to be coping very well.

DISCUSSION AND LESSONS LEARNED

- This case demonstrates the often masked presentation of alcoholism— easily missed, but so obvious in retrospect. The need to document alcohol intake accurately in the history is clearly evident.
- Dealing with an alcohol problem is not easy. Confrontation and subsequent support worked well for this patient, but it continued to be a battle, especially in view of her stoic character and the many traumatic experiences she needed to work through.

Alcoholics anonymous: two sagas

Saga 1: hot flushes

A 29-year-old married motor mechanic consulted me for the first time, complaining of episodes of facial flushing associated with 'blotchiness' of the skin of his trunk and difficulty in breathing. Sometimes he would feel very ill and eventually vomit. He said the symptoms occurred only when he drank beer, but not every time. When he drank beer he would usually smoke cigarettes. He said he was taking no medication and had no history of atopic disease. Examination was unremarkable. I told him I thought he had an allergy and considered a possible carcinoid tumour. We agreed he would take further note of his episodes and report to me.

I next saw him three months later for a ringworm infection. He said the flushing episodes had resolved spontaneously, and so we let the matter rest.

About two years later he was 'retrenched' from his job while on holiday, and his wife came to see me. She said he was drinking heavily. It emerged that he had been abusing alcohol for many years. As she described the effects of his drinking on their marriage and young family, she confided that in her desperation to help him she had on several occasions 'spiked' his coffee with disulfiram (Antabuse), obtained when he had once attended an alcohol rehabilitation program (Figure 3.2). She was aware of the link with his flushing symptoms and was surprised that I had not realised what was causing them.

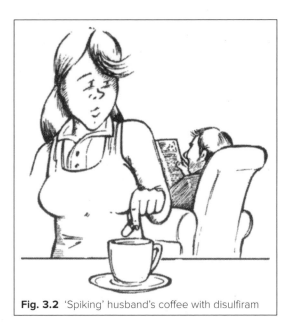

Fig. 3.2 'Spiking' husband's coffee with disulfiram

This story is a reminder that alcoholism can present in many ways: in this case, the surreptitious administration of medication by a worried family member.

Saga 2: exchanging milk for beer

George, a 49-year-old dairy farmer and former army officer, presented with gouty arthritis and dyspepsia. He had a history of hypertension, which had deteriorated in recent years.

His plethoric bloated facies and continued complaints of anxiety and insomnia made me question him carefully about his alcohol intake. 'I have only a glass or two a day, Doc. It's not a big deal: ask the wife and the boys at the pub and the RSL club,' was George's emphatic reply.

With time and a steady rise in his blood pressure, plethora and anxiety, and a continuing decline in his general health and libido, I strongly suspected a considerable intake of alcohol. I checked his story with his wife and the 'boys' at the local hotel. They confirmed his relatively sober habits.

Eventually George developed a cardiac arrhythmia and had to be admitted to hospital. His convalescence provided his bemused visitors with a somewhat convincing swatting of spiders on his bed with his slippers and description of the non-existent circus parading through the town. George and his family continued to deny the alcohol problem: 'Get off the bandwagon for God's sake—I have only the odd one,' he said.

One day, while treating the milk-tanker driver, I casually asked him how many bottles of beer he delivered to George. After an uncomfortable pause, the expected revelation was made: 'A dozen large bottles every other morning'.

The outcome was eventually positive. With the help of Alcoholics Anonymous, George managed to control his addiction and now enjoys better health but I remained concerned.

DISCUSSION AND LESSONS LEARNED

- As general practitioners we have a golden opportunity and considerable responsibility to detect alcohol and other drug abuse. We should be prepared to back our clinical judgement and diplomatically confront our patients about the problem when it arises.

- It is difficult if patients use denial or fabrication to hide a drinking problem. They will go to extraordinary lengths—including bribery—to conceal it from their families and friends.

Zoster—the 'red face' condition

Why do we often refer to herpes zoster (shingles) as one of the pitfalls or causes of a 'red face' for the general practitioner?

The reason is that it can present as pain well before the onset of the characteristic vesicular rash in the dermatome or dermatomes. It is common for two or more contiguous dermatomes to be involved especially in the thoracic dermatomes. The patient may be given an inappropriate diagnosis (often guesswork) or treatment prior to the diagnosis.

There is a prodromal or window period of about two to three weeks. Sometimes we have administered physical therapy to the spine for spinal dysfunction—quite an embarrassment! A particular diagnostic brain teaser is where only one or two maculopapular eruptions, separated by considerable space, appear in the dermatome.

Case 1

In the example shown, a 38-year-old butcher presented with a painful lump on his back adjacent to the spine. (Refer to Figure 3.3, centre insert page 2.) He said that it felt like a boil, but when his wife introduced a needle it drained only a small amount of blood and no purulent material. It was only when he was stripped of clothing and closely examined that the other two lesions were observed on the anterior chest wall. It was herpes zoster of dermatome T7.

Case 2

A 55-year-old hairdresser presented with the pain of classic right-sided sciatica involving the L5 dermatome which was not alleviated by over-the-counter analgesics. While testing her reflexes I noticed two vesicular lesions on the outside of her leg at the level of the knee. She had herpes zoster.

DISCUSSION AND LESSONS LEARNED

- In any painful unilateral presentation, consider the possibility of herpes zoster, especially in an older person. Infants can also develop herpes zoster.
- Where the cause of the pain is not obvious, search carefully in the distribution of the dermatome.
- Herpes zoster of the trigeminal nerve is common (15% of all cases) and herpes zoster ophthalmicus (involvement of the ophthalmic division) can be complex. Lesions on the tip, root and side of the nose and the inner corner of the eye indicate herpes zoster ophthalmicus and serious eye involvement can develop. Referral to an ophthalmologist may be appropriate. Sporadic lesions can occur in the scalp.
- Keep in mind the condition of 'Zoster Sine Zoster' where nerve involvement can occur without the cutaneous rash. Tricky!
- A delay in the diagnosis of herpes zoster (shingles) and/or failure to prescribe antiviral medication in a timely manner can be a cause of complaints and claims against GPs where the patient develops post-herpetic neuralgia.

Not in the script

It was during consulting hours on the Australia Day holiday that the receptionist for our group practice contacted me saying, 'I have a gentleman who doesn't want to see you but insists on a prescription for Ventolin. Could you oblige?'

The practice rule is not to prescribe without seeing the patient. When I left my consulting room I noticed a very formidable, impatient character pacing around looking rather like a Hereford bull waiting for springtime—massive, plethoric, humourless and with a RAAF-like moustache. He was an arrogant 56-year-old business executive.

His confrontation was incisive and threatening: 'Bloggs of Bentleigh, Doc. I just want a script of Ventolin for my asthma—haven't got time to wait around'. Despite my feelings of annoyance I thought it expedient to follow the soft option and I quickly scribbled a script for the simple anti-asthmatic drug.

Three months later on Easter Saturday, the receptionist informed me that a man was at her desk wanting a repeat of his 'blood pressure pills'. It was Bloggs, who reluctantly agreed to my insistence that he should wait to be seen. In swaggered Bloggs—fidgety, very plethoric, obese, the sound of wheezing punctuating his laboured alcohol-saturated breath, uncomfortable about his subordinate role.

'I've had this asthma on and off for two years ever since you fellows changed my blood pressure tablets.' As I perused his history the answer became painfully obvious.

Diagnosis

Two years previously the patient's antihypertensive therapy was altered when metoprolol was substituted for methyldopa. At the same time the attending doctor stressed the importance of reducing weight, smoking and alcohol intake. The change to a beta blocker precipitated bronchial asthma, which had been quiescent since his adolescence.

DISCUSSION AND LESSONS LEARNED

- The beta blocker had been prescribed without careful consideration of the past history of asthma.
- To achieve compliance and better management, careful follow up should have been emphasised with specific times given for review.
- It is important that consistent strict rules should apply for repeat prescriptions, especially for antihypertensives, and clear guidelines given to the reception staff. Special care should be taken with manipulative patients: their evasiveness may indicate another problem such as alcoholism.

Perplexing chest pain

Case 1

Marge T, aged 52, presented with an extraordinary story of modern medical mismanagement. While carrying heavy suitcases in Hong Kong, she developed anterior chest pain. She was taken to an emergency department where, despite a normal ECG, she was told she had heart trouble and had to be careful.

Upon returning to Melbourne and while under the care of her son-in-law, who was a specialist, she developed episodes of central chest pain with, at times, mid-thoracic back pain. She felt tired and languid. A stress ECG was normal. She was admitted to a teaching hospital for further investigation. Unfortunately, an ultrasound examination was reported to be abnormal (? chronic relapsing pancreatitis). The incompatible clinical history was ignored as she went from investigation to investigation over a period of nine months. The eventual diagnosis was chest pain of unknown cause with anxiety.

Diagnosis and outcome

As a result, the anxious and devastated Marge first consulted me with classic depression. The history was interesting—the pain invariably followed a lifting or laborious activity such as vacuuming and bed-making. The associated back pain tended to get ignored as the focus was on the retrosternal pain. Examination revealed tenderness at the T5 and T6 levels of her thoracic spine while a plain X-ray showed mild degenerative changes.

She had dysfunction of her mid-thoracic spine with referred pain. After three treatments by spinal mobilisation and manipulation, her pain completely subsided as did her 'stress-related problem', anxiety and depression (although it took some months).

Case 2

Elana W, aged 32, presented as a new patient with epigastric pain brought on by physical activity including lifting her children. A careful history determined associated back pain 'just around my bra strap'. The problematic T7 area of her thoracic spine was appropriately treated.

Elana came in with one of her children some weeks later and said, 'You know, Doctor, that stomach pain I've had for three years has gone. To think that it was thought to be an ulcer and then a hiatus hernia. I've had two barium meals and a tube passed down, but they found nothing.'

Case 3

Joan G, aged 41, requested a second opinion about recurrent pains under her right costal margin for 12 months or so. Cholecystectomy did not help at all, but correction of her thoracic spinal problem at T7–T8 completely alleviated the pain.

Case 4

The author has a personal testimony worth recording. Poliomyelitis affected the back at 8 years of age; from age 12 to 24 persistent thoracic back pain would radiate antero-laterally just below the nipple line, either right or left side. 'You have to learn to live with it John—it will probably get worse as you get older', came the reassuring prognostication from my attending neurologist.

Other more adventurous doctors proffered diagnoses such as post-polio neuralgia, Da Costa's syndrome and Tietze's syndrome. I noted during medical school that if patients were unfortunate enough to get the pain on the left side of the chest it was called 'cardiac neurosis'.

However, while attending a football club physiotherapist for an ankle injury, he noted my thoracic deformity and asked if it gave me pain, saying, 'I can fix that.' 'No, you can't,' I responded. 'Yes, I can—let me try.' Thumbs and hands deftly worked on the T4–T6 levels—impressive sound effects with cracking and clicking. To the profound relief and gratitude of this impressionable patient, the 13 years of pain was relieved. Yes, it returns occasionally but is likewise fixed with physical therapy.

DISCUSSION AND LESSONS LEARNED

- The medical profession tends to have a blind spot with various pain syndromes in the chest, especially the anterior chest and upper abdomen, caused by the common problem of dysfunction of the thoracic spine.

- Doctors who gain this insight are amazed at how often they diagnose the cause that previously did not enter their 'programmed' medical minds.
- Physical therapy to the spine can be dramatically effective when used appropriately. Unfortunately, many of us associate it with quackery. It was an interesting experience presenting Marge T's case to a grand round at one of the hospitals who mismanaged her. The consultants were divided in their responses. Many accepted the insight with knowing gratitude while others became very upset and threatened.
- It is devastating for patients to create doubts in their minds about having a 'heart problem' or an 'anxiety neurosis'. Substituting vague or even dogmatic incorrect labels for ignorance is a dishonest strategy.

A classic golden trap

Molly W, aged 78, came in with her shopping list of symptoms, one of the 'heartsinks' of a frantically busy practice. With slow, monotonous deliberation she reeled off the problems. 'I feel sick, Doctor—you know nauseous, not myself, no energy, off my food, constipated, headachey, sore in the back, sore tummy, no get-up-and-go, not sleeping well, everything is an effort, I get thirsty and I tire out easily.'

'Typical general practice problem,' I mused, 'undifferentiated illness—epidemic proportions this week.' Could she be hypothyroid? Polymyalgia rheumatica? Anaemia? No, she must be depressed with a history like that.

Diagnosis and outcome

I ordered haemoglobin, blood film, ESR, random blood sugar and thyroid function tests. All these tests were normal. Upon review she said that she felt much the same, but the anorexia and nausea had increased and she felt hot and clammy. I was convinced that she was depressed, but I remembered to attend to a routine that I overlooked on the first visit—an office test of the urine. To my surprise (and relief) it showed positive to protein, blood and nitrite. Microscopy of the urine showed copious pus cells and bacteria. All her symptoms had virtually abated two days after commencing antibiotics.

DISCUSSION AND LESSONS LEARNED

- Despite being 'bitten' many times, one continues to be fooled by the urinary infection, especially in the elderly and in children. Typical symptoms such as dysuria and frequency may be absent or not offered as complaints.
- The importance of routine office testing of the urine in such cases is obvious. Many general practitioners insist that their unwell patients bring a specimen of urine each time they come to the office.
- All general practitioners without ready access to pathology services should have a microscope and be proficient in its use to examine urine in suspected urinary infection.
- Undifferentiated illness is a common problem presenting in general practice and it requires a plan of management. Typical causes are depression, diabetes mellitus, drugs (iatrogenic or self-administered), anaemia, hypothyroidism, malignant disease and urinary tract infection.
- A 'quick fix' answer to undifferentiated illness is very difficult in a busy general practice with the pressure of 'wall-to-wall patients'. Critics do not appreciate how difficult it can be, especially with some 'heartsink' patients.

Tales of *Campylobacter jejuni*

Annie

Annie, a 23-year-old secretary, presented with a three-day history of diarrhoea with blood and mucus, abdominal pain and general malaise. A diarrhoeal illness two months before had settled spontaneously, with normal bowel action up until the latest presentation. Her history was unremarkable apart from appendicectomy. She was on the oral contraceptive pill. In particular, there was no other bowel disturbance or family history of bowel disease. A general examination showed a relatively fit person with a soft abdomen and a rectal examination revealed soft stool. Sigmoidoscopy to 10 cm showed an inflamed, ulcerated rectum with some contact bleeding.

In view of the severity of proctitis and concern of ulcerative colitis, urgent gastroenterological referral was organised. The consultant's diagnosis was ulcerative colitis. Biopsies were taken and sulfasalazine commenced. The biopsies were consistent with ulcerative colitis.

Nausea and persistent malaise on sulfasalazine prompted a change to mesalazine. Fortunately stool cultures had been obtained by the gastroenterologist and *Campylobacter jejuni* was cultured. Mesalazine was ceased and azithromycin prescribed. Subsequently all symptoms settled, much to the patient's joy and her doctor's relief.

Kay

Kay U, a 29-year-old mother of two young children, presented 10 days after Annie. She had a longstanding history of ulcerative colitis. She had experienced numerous (two to three per year) severe flare-ups requiring high-dose oral and local corticosteroids with ongoing maintenance with sulfasalazine. She presented with what appeared to be a further exacerbation with abdominal pain, diarrhoea with blood and mucus. She commenced oral prednisolone (30 mg per day) and rectal hydrocortisone. However, her symptoms did not improve and contact with her gastroenterologist prompted further increase of the oral corticosteroid.

Persistent failure of her symptoms to improve prompted the gastroenterologist to request admission to our local country hospital for high doses of intravenous hydrocortisone and bedrest with nil orally. Fortunately, in view of our recent experience with Annie and despite Kay's well-known ulcerative colitis, he advised us to organise stool cultures.

After several days of high-dose steroid, the patient had some significant improvement in stool function and was feeling significantly better and desperately hungry. Stool cultures paradoxically were positive for *Campylobacter jejuni* and azithromycin was prescribed and steroids reduced. Fortunately again, stool function returned to normal.

DISCUSSION AND LESSONS LEARNED

These case histories serve to highlight the reality that *Campylobacter* can masquerade as an acute proctitis as part of an ulcerative colitis. It certainly outlines the necessity when faced with acute proctitis to think of *Campylobacter* infection. The occurrence in a patient with ongoing ulcerative colitis is a concern. I suppose the clue here was the failure of the patient to respond to her normally successful self-medication.

Endocrine tales

Chapter 4

> *It would indeed be rash for a mere pathologist to venture*
> *forth on the uncharted sea of the endocrines, strewn as it is*
> *with the wrecks of shattered hypotheses, where even the most*
> *wary mariner may easily lose his way as he seeks to steer*
> *his bark amid the glandular temptations whose siren voices*
> *have proved the downfall of many who have gone before.*

William Boyd (1885–1969)

Death without a diagnosis for chronic fatigue

This classic cautionary case about a 16-year-old Western Australian female student serves as a reminder that any of us could be misled by the capricious Addison's disease. She presented to her general practitioner with four weeks of fatigue and tiredness. Her mother reported that she suffered from malaise and anorexia and had lost weight and seemed prone to 'pick up any bugs that were going around'. There was no significant past history although she was reportedly diagnosed as having glandular fever six months previously. Physical examination was normal. A series of blood tests, including a full blood examination, was ordered and reported as normal.

Over the next four to five months the patient continued to feel unwell and stopped attending school because she felt so tired and lacked energy for her usual activities including sport. Other reported problems included poor concentration, somnolence, continued loss of weight, anorexia, vomiting (up to five times a week) and syncope during venesection followed by prolonged dizziness. She had several consultations with different practitioners including a mental health assessment but was still without a firm diagnosis. Physical examinations were recorded as 'unremarkable' despite a discussion, probably initiated by her father, about skin colour changes.

During her final blood test at the GP's clinic she fainted and remained too dizzy to return home. She was referred to the local hospital for resuscitation with intravenous fluids. Back at home she remained unwell but refused her parents' wish to attend for review of her blood tests. Her parents were in the process of taking the by now rather cachexic girl to hospital when she was found dead in bed. The post-mortem examination concluded that the cause of death was adrenal insufficiency due to autoimmune destruction of the adrenal cortex (Bird, 2007a).

More medical brain teasers

- I recall seeing a 7-year-old boy in the emergency department of the Children's Hospital referred from a physician in a provincial city because of two months of dizzy spells and blackouts. I performed a routine blood sugar and found hypoglycaemia. The penny dropped. I went looking for and found hyperpigmentation in the oral mucosa.

- Recently I received an email from a British GP saying that it took two and a half years for her Addison's disease to be diagnosed. Another member of the UK Addison's Disease Self Help Group waited 15 years to be diagnosed after treatment for depression and chronic fatigue syndrome. A 9-year-old child with asthma from three years of age was eventually diagnosed with secondary Addison's disease after ten hospital admissions in five years for recurrent vomiting and diarrhoea. The writer was sympathetic to the difficulty of diagnosis and pointed out that the single blood tests were unreliable. 'Highlight it in your books' was the message.

- A friend developed diarrhoea during a stressful trip to Nepal (having accidents and being robbed). Two weeks of lethargy, anorexia, nausea, vomiting, diarrhoea and abdominal pain followed. She was then treated with Flagyl for presumed giardiasis. After collapsing at home, she was admitted to hospital confused, febrile and hypotensive. Four days after being discharged to home, she collapsed again and was readmitted to hospital semi-conscious. This was diagnosed as an Addisonian crisis. Her eventual outcome has been good.

DISCUSSION AND LESSONS LEARNED

- Addison's disease (primary adrenal insufficiency) is another of the classic great pretenders and is notoriously difficult to diagnose in its early stages.
- As GPs we need to be highly suspicious of this disease when a condition remains undiagnosed. Consider it in patients with any of the following: excessive fatigue, anorexia/nausea/vomiting, abdominal pain, weight loss, dizziness/funny turns/postural hypotension.
- Look for hyperpigmentation especially of the mucous membranes of the mouth and hard palate, and skin creases of the hands. It may be a late feature.
- Avoid using the phrase 'the physical examination was unremarkable'.
- Use the 'baseball rule'—three strikes and you're out! Get another opinion.

A lighter shade of pale

Gladys was a delightful 81-year-old lady, who had been attending for 12 years with angina pectoris and mild congestive cardiac failure. The latter had been well controlled with the daily administration of digoxin 0.125 mg, chlorothiazide 0.5 g and potassium chloride 1200 mg. She was taking glyceryl trinitrate (nitroglycerin) for her angina.

Then one day she presented with increasing dyspnoea on exertion, weakness and nocturia. The diagnosis of poorly controlled congestive cardiac failure was made, and frusemide 80 mg with increased potassium was added to her daily regimen. The serum digoxin level ordered at this visit was normal.

She improved slowly but on review was still weak and short of breath. I noticed that she was pale and frail but otherwise appeared normal for her age. The results of further blood tests were as follows:

Haemoglobin	102 g/L (115–165 g/L)
PCV (packed cell volume)	33% (36–48%)
Normochromic normocytic anaemia	
ESR	48
Platelets and WCC	normal

In view of her age I rationalised that as her anaemia was mild no further investigations were warranted. Furthermore, I considered that no likely treatable cause would be found. I placed her on isosorbide nitrate, iron tablets and multivitamins with a reassurance that she would cope nicely if she took 'things easy'.

Diagnosis

During my holiday leave Gladys presented with a severe episode of angina, and she was treated by my GP registrar who decided to investigate her problem further. He ordered thyroid function tests, blood glucose, urea and electrolytes. Upon my return the pathology slip waiting in my pigeon hole read as follows:

Serum thyroxine (free T4) 3.4 (8–22 pmol/L)
Serum TSH (thyroid-stimulating hormone) 91.9 (0.4–5.5 uU/mL)

She was hypothyroid, thus providing the answer for her normochromic anaemia and her medical dysequilibrium. This fact was not clinically obvious to us.

DISCUSSION AND LESSONS LEARNED

- Elderly patients can be a reservoir of unexpected surprises and clinical traps, often because we tend to manage them superficially and rationalise their deterioration in health as an integral part of the ageing process. They deserve the same analytical thinking about their malaise as younger patients.

- The common problems requiring frequent attendance and skilful therapeutic management are ischaemic heart disease and congestive cardiac failure.
- If an unexplained deterioration occurs in a patient with congestive cardiac failure we should think about digitalis (now rarely used) toxicity, hypokalaemia or anaemia. However, thyroid disease is more common than appreciated and is one of the great 'masquerades'. Gladys, like so many patients in general practice, showed no obvious signs of the disease. She was thin with a normal pulse and facial appearance, but she did have dry skin and some hair loss that I considered normal for her age. My final mistake was not to take the investigations to their logical end point. Incidentally, Gladys felt 'much younger' once taking thyroxine.

Missing links

The words 'missing links' may bring to mind thoughts on evolution, apes, near-humans and the origin of the species. But in day-to-day medical practice missing links can be the cause of significant and serious medical conditions. These links, or factors, when discovered and put back into place will bring about the reversal of all, or most, ill effects caused by the absence of that vital link and make a sick person healthy.

The effects and changes caused by the missing factors may be insidious, may take a long time to reveal obvious clinical signs, are easily missed and often embarrass the unwary observer. The resulting conditions may come to light in people that you know well and see frequently, and who have complete faith in your capabilities and clinical acumen.

Now the stories unfold . . .

Mrs S

Mrs S, in her fifties, had not had a comfortable life. She had nine children, not all of them easy to manage, and had become a grandmother at an early age with added caring responsibilities. Her husband had always been a heavy drinker and at an early age developed Parkinson's disease, with total incapacity.

Understandably, I thought, she always seemed to be tired, to have difficulty with her weight and to be depressed. Because of her various involvements, I saw Mrs S frequently and sympathised with her feelings and predicament. I failed to notice that she felt the cold easily, and that her voice was getting deeper and her hair coarser. It was not until I noticed her change in features from Mrs Jekyll to Mrs Hyde that the penny dropped. Appropriate investigations and correct treatment quickly followed. The thyroxine worked like magic, and we saw the return of the Mrs S we all used to know. Myxoedema can trap even the experienced observer.

On a visit to Mrs S several months later I thought her features were a bit coarse, and she said she had been having weight problems again. A check on her thyroid function tests showed that her thyroid needs had increased. Be ever watchful.

Laura

Sometimes the illness caused by the missing link can be life threatening, suddenly and dramatically.

Laura was a 13-year-old, full of energy and a strong tennis player. She was one of three children in a happy family. Her brother, three years older, had been blind from birth and had become epileptic at an early age. Laura presented on a Monday afternoon with persistent vomiting, and as there was a lot of vomiting of viral aetiology in children of the district she was diagnosed as having viral gastroenteritis. Her condition did not improve and I saw her on Friday of that same week. As we went carefully over the history I could not help but notice that Laura was falling asleep upright in the chair, ready to topple over.

'How long has she been like this?'

'Only today.'

'Has she been passing much urine?'

'She never seems to stop.'

'Before the vomiting episode, was she drinking a lot?'

'We kept running out of soft drink, cordial and fruit juice.'

'Had she been well?'

'She's been very tired—she couldn't even be bothered with her beloved tennis.'

A quick blood sugar test showed a sky-high level; a ketotic Laura was admitted to hospital that afternoon. By Monday morning she was back home, well and self-injecting with insulin twice daily. She was her old self, having accepted her missing link philosophically.

As we know, when the particular factor or link goes missing in such cases as myxoedema, diabetes mellitus, pernicious anaemia and Addison's disease, we have a serious, life-threatening, often insidious disease evolving. The recognition of the missing link and its immediate replacement will bring about a miraculous recovery that has the patient saying, 'Doctor, I've never felt better in my life'.

DISCUSSION AND LESSONS LEARNED

- There are common conditions that occur because of a missing link in our complicated biochemical mechanisms, and that present as beautiful clinical entities before a vigilant observer.

- Every day in our patient contacts there may be a missing link for us to discover and identify and we must do our utmost to ensure that we never miss that vital link.

- 10 to 70 per cent of children at the onset of type 1 diabetes mellitus present in diabetic ketoacidosis. A systematic review (Usher-Smith, 2011) found that children presenting with diabetic ketoacidosis had symptoms for a mean of two weeks, and up to a third had at least one medical consultation in the week before diagnosis. Patients with diabetic ketoacidosis usually present with polyuria, polydipsia, polyphagia, fatigue and weakness and Kussmaul's respirations; nausea and vomiting are present in 50–80 per cent of patients and abdominal pain is present in about 30 per cent.

- High rates of misdiagnosis have also been found in children presenting with type 1 diabetes without diabetic ketoacidosis, with up to 86 per cent of children not diagnosed at first encounter. Common diagnostic errors include misinterpreting symptoms (such as polyuria misdiagnosed as urinary tract infection); exclusively focusing on one or more symptoms (such as oral candidiasis); and not performing appropriate investigations (such as blood glucose or urine tests).

An overactive thyroid and an underactive cerebral cortex

Mrs Leyma K, a recently arrived Latvian immigrant, presented with an English-speaking cousin. Leyma could not communicate in English at all. Her cousin said that she wanted Leyma to have a good check-up and would like her to be referred to a multiphasic screening centre. Leyma had felt uncharacteristically nervous and irritable since her arrival in Australia four months ago.

Leyma had visited a Latvian-speaking doctor who was very abrupt with her and prescribed a benzodiazepine for an anxiety state, but apparently she felt worse on the tranquiliser.

I was rushed and so I took a brief history via the interpreter, who said that Leyma was feeling stressed and upset about leaving her native country and was finding the heat of the Australian summer unbearable. I wrote out a referral to the screening centre.

Two weeks later I received a most impressive and expensive computer print-out with one abnormal test among the hundreds. Her thyroid function tests showed marked hyperthyroidism. The diagnosis had been staring me in the face: thin, anxious, sweaty, tachycardiac and intolerant to heat although no eye signs.

DISCUSSION AND LESSONS LEARNED
- We tend to get distracted by the language communication barrier when we should not, and we sometimes take short cuts when more attention to detail would clinch the diagnosis.
- I have to confess to being fooled by thyrotoxicosis masquerading as an anxiety state on many occasions. I now have a working rule that 'thyrotoxicosis has to be excluded in an apparent anxiety state'.
- The outstanding presenting part of our patients is the face, which is certainly a 'mirror of disease'. As general practitioners, we have to

discipline ourselves to read all the clues from our patient's physical features and body language.

- We can be easily misled by circumstantial factors, for example abnormal stress causing the problem, especially when it represents the easy option for the busy doctor.
- We should avoid referral to multiphasic screening centres and be more discriminating and specific in the tests that we order.

The 'bomb happy' soldier

During the full fury of the Pacific War in 1943 the army discharged Eddie Murphy, a 32-year-old soldier, back to the care of his general practitioner. Apparently Eddie had become sick during action; he felt very irritable, nervous and weak, and was hospitalised for four months with a short spell in the 'bomb happy' ward.

Eddie's problem baffled the doctors, including a panel of three consultants who detected an abnormality with his heart rhythm. They concluded eventually that Eddie's problem was functional and gave him an honourable discharge with the diagnosis of 'disordered action of the heart'.

His GP was amazed to find that Eddie looked ill, was rather agitated and had lost weight. When he shook Eddie's hand and instinctively felt his pulse, the diagnosis was obvious.

Diagnosis and outcome

Eddie had thyrotoxicosis—rather classic apart from the lack of exophthalmos. His warm sweaty palms and atrial fibrillation were very significant. However, in making this diagnosis his GP enjoyed the distinct advantage of already having treated two members of his family with the same problem. Fortunately, Eddie responded nicely to a prolonged course of iodine in milk and spent the duration of the war in 'active service' on his farm.

Sleeping sickness

One Sunday morning a person rang urgently to say that her 78-year-old mother-in-law, Mrs Williams, who had arrived to stay, was very ill. 'Would you please call, Doctor?' she said. I initially baulked at the prospect, because the caller had moved out of my area to a suburb some 8 km away. The elderly patient's doctor, whose surgery was only 5 km away, refused to call because it was outside his 2 km 'call limit'.

However, I continued to listen. 'It is not possible to rouse mother for breakfast. She is in a coma, Doctor. She was discharged from hospital yesterday after convalescing from a total hip replacement. She has had a wound infection but she seemed quite well last night. She has a bottle with some Serepax in it by her bed.'

The mind started racing. 'Why should I go? An overdose—great! I'll call an ambulance. No, I'll get her doctor to go—no, I'll call her surgeon.' These escapist thoughts were interrupted by a persuasive interjection, 'Could you please help us—we don't know what to do'.

'Damn—I'll go,' I thought. 'It's probably a cerebrovascular accident (CVA) anyway or septicaemia. Myocardial infarction? Pulmonary embolus? No, most likely an overdose—the lady's depressed or confused.'

With the adrenaline running high, I arrived at the house. The anxious relatives looked relieved. I was led into a cold, damp room to find a semiconscious elderly woman lying in bed. (Refer to Figure 4.1, centre insert page 2.) She would respond to painful stimuli by throwing her arms about and moaning. There were no neurological abnormalities on physical examination.

Temperature was 36.5 °C (*per axilla*), pulse 86/min, respiratory rate 16/min, blood pressure 160/90. What could the problem be?

I could not really tell if she had overdosed on Serepax. I searched and found a bottle of glibenclamide (Daonil) tablets in her handbag.

'Could she have hypoglycaemia? Well probably not—that's usually caused by insulin,' I thought.

In my doctor's bag, I found a bottle of Dextrostix. Two months beyond expiry date. I wished I had my glucometer with me. However, I took some blood from her fingertip (provoking a response) and tested it—3 mmol/L.

Now to impress everyone! I checked for a suitable vein (which was present), seized a vial of 50 per cent dextrose solution, drew the contents into a 20 mL syringe and injected the rather cumbersome solution. Within a minute the real Mrs Williams awoke and looked around the room bemused, especially at the stranger who stood over her looking pleased.

I was certainly glad I went on that house call. I love diagnosing and treating hypoglycaemic attacks. It's one of the few times a general practitioner feels really powerful and satisfied.

It brought back recent memories of being called to Cyril, an elderly diabetic, who was found unconscious on the floor of the local supermarket. The curious crowd thought he was stone dead and he certainly looked it. Imagine the reaction when this 'corpse' sat up as large as life when 'the treacle' was injected by the apparently calm, all-knowing GP. Even the anti-doctor critics were impressed.

DISCUSSION AND LESSONS LEARNED

- Hypoglycaemia should certainly be considered in any patient, unknown to us, who is found to be unconscious. A golden rule is: 'In the absence of trauma, the unconscious patient has hypoglycaemia until proved otherwise'.
- We should be mindful that oral hypoglycaemic agents can cause hypoglycaemic coma, especially if patients double up their dosage!

- It is worth having fresh 'strips' in the doctor's bag to measure blood sugar, albeit an estimate. It is also important to carry 50 per cent dextrose or glucagon in the doctor's bag. A more practical approach is to give glucagon 1 mL intramuscularly followed by a sugary drink and/or sweets.
- A quick phone call to the patient's regular doctor is advisable if possible.
- Searching for every conceivable clue to assist the diagnosis is most important. A check for illness identification on the patient is recommended.
- Home visits for emergency situations are important, very rewarding and most appreciated by the community.

A bronze medal

Mrs Fraser, a farmer's wife, came to me with a minor ailment not long after she moved with her husband and two children to the district. She brought with her a letter, written by their previous family doctor in South Australia, which informed me that her husband was a type 1 diabetic.

Shortly after harvest Mr Fraser came in to renew his insulin prescription. Tall, slim, tanned and seemingly very healthy, he was a pleasant man and well educated in the management and possible complications of his disease. Most of our consultation was devoted to discussion of general topics. His file already had been marked 'diabetic' and I looked forward to having little to do for him except write his insulin prescriptions. (The days of glycosylated haemoglobin and glucometers were yet to come.)

Four months later he consulted me for the second and last time. He said he had felt 'off colour' for two or three months and so had been taking some of his wife's iron tablets left over from her last pregnancy. Now he felt generally unwell and noticed his ankles were swollen.

Examination revealed that he was in cardiac failure. Then the penny dropped: his tan was not a 'healthy suntan' but bronzing. He had haemochromatosis, a rarity but something that should have occurred to me when I first saw him.

My preconception that he had diabetes was a misconception.

LESSON LEARNED

If a bird flies in your window it probably is a sparrow but it could be a canary: if you do not recognise the possibility you might not see the bird for what it is.

Diabetes with a difference

Harold, a 57-year-old builder, had been a patient of mine for 25 years. He had a history of peripheral neuropathy of unknown cause, controlled by exchange transfusion with immunoglobulin. In 1962 he acquired syphilis with no apparent sequelae. He smoked 30 cigarettes per day and was a teetotaller.

In August 1990, a random glucose was 5 mmol/L but in September 1991, when a blood lipid profile was ordered, a random glucose was 10 mmol/L, while random cholesterol was only 3.7 mmol/L and triglycerides was 5.9 mmol/L.

A fasting glucose, which was then ordered, was 6 mmol/L. Although these figures did not satisfy the criteria for diagnosis of diabetes (7 mmol/L fasting or 11 mmol/L random), I was suspicious about the possibility and ordered a glucose tolerance test.

This showed a fasting glucose of 20, a 1 hour of 32.5 and 2 hours of 35 mmol/L. Insulin was 13, 11 and 17 units respectively. All insulins were within the normal range.

He was diagnosed as a type 2 diabetic. He was started on a diet with the help of a diabetic educator and his blood sugar level (BSL) was monitored.

He was most cooperative, and his weight decreased from 72 kg to 59 kg and his BSL remained constantly in the normal range.

Abdominal mass

In May 1992 he noticed a lump in his abdomen. Examination disclosed a pulsating lump and a CT scan showed a small abdominal aortic aneurysm.

The CT, which was repeated in September 1992, showed no changes in the size of the aneurysm and no other abnormality in the abdominal organs. Harold continued to lose weight and although this was a concern to me it was attributed to his zealous dieting.

His height was 171.5 cm and with a weight of 59 kg that represents a body mass index of 20, just inside the normal of 20 to 25.

In November 1992 he complained of right upper quadrant abdominal pain. He was tender but not jaundiced. Liver function tests showed normal bilirubin and alkaline phosphatase but the aspartate transaminase (AST formerly SGOT) was slightly raised at 75 units (normal, 60). The pain and tenderness settled without treatment while a follow-up AST was 2 units.

Harold requested a repeat CT of his abdomen in January 1993. The CT was reported as follows: 'In the scans throughout the upper abdomen there are multiple low-density lesions present in the liver, the appearance suggests metastatic disease. The head of the pancreas appears a little irregular, the appearance is not marked but in view of the liver findings a carcinoma would have to be considered'.

At laparotomy there was a firm hard mass in the head of the pancreas with multiple liver secondaries.

Harold died in May 1993.

DISCUSSION AND LESSONS LEARNED
- The cause of his diabetes thus became evident at laparotomy.
- Common things are common.
- However, the uncommon, which may be associated with common, lies in wait for the unwary.

Insulin stopwork

A 34-year-old woman with type 1 diabetes mellitus since the age of 14 presented with a three-day history of sore throat, nausea, vomiting and chest pain radiating to the shoulder. The patient was not eating and was advised to stop taking insulin. Antibiotics were prescribed for the throat infection.

Twenty-four hours later her condition had deteriorated with persistent nausea and vomiting; in addition she was very thirsty and had polyuria. She was sent to the emergency department of a large city hospital for investigation and management.

On examination, the patient was conscious but dehydrated. Her vital signs were blood pressure 110/60, respiratory rate 22 per minute, pulse 110 per minute, temperature 36.5 °C. Urinalysis showed 110 mg glucose and large amounts of ketones. Her throat was inflamed, but there was no lymphadenopathy. A chest X-ray was normal. The provisional diagnosis was diabetic ketoacidosis.

Biochemistry

The results of serum analysis showed glucose 45 mmol/L, pH 7.24, HCO_3 11 mmol/L, Na 128 mmol/L, PO_2 110 mm Hg and PCO_2 26 mm Hg, K^+ 5.3 mmol/L, urea 8.3 mmol/L, creatinine 13 mmol/L.

Management and outcome

Intravenous normal saline (NS) was commenced to correct the dehydration at the rate of 1 L over two hours. Insulin was given by intravenous infusion—100 units of short-acting insulin (Actrapid) in 500 mL of Haemacel. The infusion rate was regulated on a sliding scale according to blood glucose levels, following a loading dose of 6 units of Actrapid, with the aim of slowly lowering the blood glucose to 7 to 10 mmol/L.

Potassium (K^+) replacement was given once urine output was established to maintain a level between 4 and 5 mmol/L. Intravenous fluid was changed to 4 per cent dextrose in NS when her blood glucose was 12 mmol/L and ceased in 24 hours—after symptoms settled and the patient was eating and drinking.

The patient was discharged five days after admission on her usual dose of insulin: Actrapid HM 8 units morning, 4 units evening and Protophane HM 18 units morning, 4 units evening. Diabetes education and management of sick days were reviewed during admission.

DISCUSSION AND LESSONS LEARNED

- Diabetic ketoacidosis is a largely preventable complication of type 1 diabetes mellitus in diagnosed patients.
- Insulin should not be stopped during illness (even if the patient is not eating) to prevent the formation of ketone bodies.
- Vomiting and nausea can be the result of ketone formation.
- Education about appropriate care during illness is essential, and the patient's knowledge of this should be reviewed.
- Increased amounts of insulin are often necessary during illness, in which case the insulin dose should be reviewed after recovery and readjusted if necessary to prevent hypoglycaemia.
- Gastric stasis and inhalation of vomitus is a possible complication of ketoacidosis, even in a conscious patient.

The last rites: 12 years premature!

I inherited the miserable Olive M, a 73-year-old mother of ten children, from my predecessor when I entered country practice. The diagnosis on the white card read 'generally worn out and depressed' and she was prescribed a tonic and thyroid extract, after a failed trial of 'purple hearts'.

Olive, who looked old, thin and depressed, would shuffle into the consulting room saying, 'I'm still a bag of misery, Doctor, I ache all over, my legs ache, especially the shins, my back aches, I've no energy and I can't eat, but the worst thing is this constipation. I get bound up and it causes gripes in my stomach. What's the point of going on like this?'

Medical school had not prepared me for this—I had heard all about 'undifferentiated illness' in general practice. There was no doubt she was depressed. Previous investigation showed normal thyroid function, full blood examination and many other tests including serum electrolytes. The only abnormality was in renal function with mildly elevated serum urea and creatinine but not in the renal failure range. Apart from a blood pressure (BP) of 180/95 there was absolutely nothing abnormal to find on the physical examination.

I stopped the thyroid extract and prescribed antidepressants. When I followed up with a house call, I found her in bed behaving irrationally and complaining of generalised itching. She was psychotic and she kept saying that she 'was ready to meet the Lord'. I then admitted her to hospital.

Diagnosis and outcome

When I arrived for my usual evening rounds I found the priest giving her the last rites. The family had all assembled. One of the sons who had some peripheral medical knowledge had decided Mum was dying and her death was imminent, despite my prognostications that this was not so and that 'we would get to the bottom of it'.

In frustration I decided to ring a colleague who had just passed his physician's exams and was an excellent diagnostician, especially with the rare and obscure. After listening to the history Roger said it all with just a few well-chosen words: 'John, moans, bones and abdominal groans—remember? Any stones?' Within a few weeks Olive had her parathyroid adenoma removed by a skilled neck surgeon in Melbourne. The transformation was incredible. A normal, happy, energetic and wonderful woman would see me and tell me how clever I was. I informed her that if I had been clever I would have saved her three months of moans, bones, abdominal groans, constipation and humiliation.

Olive died 12 years later. As the priest with his delightful Irish wit said, 'Can't beat the last rites, works wonders!'

DISCUSSION AND LESSONS LEARNED

- There is something about our healing art that keeps us humble or should do so.
- Endocrine disorders—in addition to neurological problems—can be the real brain-teasers in general practice. One can only hope that one does not miss the diagnosis when a similar problem reappears.
- Most people can be delightful, energetic and normal when we cure their disease. We have a God-given responsibility to 'find the real person'.

Too big for their boots

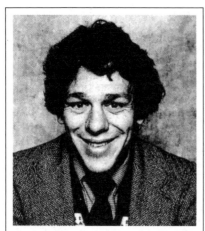

Fig. 4.2 Mike (1 year before diagnosis)

'Did you see cousin Mike at the family funeral?'

'No, I didn't see him.'

'Well you wouldn't recognise him. He looks strange, as though there's something wrong with his glands,' came the layperson's reply.

Then I recalled seeing a fellow who looked acromegalic. Further inquiries revealed that the acromegalic-looking 'stranger' at the funeral was indeed the unrecognisable Mike, a 38-year-old teacher (Figure 4.2).

A phone call to his concerned mother determined that Mike had been unwell for seven years, but at the moment was having radiological investigation through his general practitioner who, at last, had heard a 'penny drop'. The saga for Mike was remarkable. For the past seven years his mother had observed him becoming 'bigger and uglier'. He was noticed to become very tired, irritable and sweaty.

A discussion with Mike produced a very interesting version. The first thing he noticed was broadening and enlarging of his nose, which was subject to two operations by an ENT surgeon. Over a period of six years he noticed also the following symptoms and signs that developed slowly:

- clothing became tighter, especially shirts with buttons
- hands increased in size and became thicker
- 'pimples' (almost like boils) appeared on his back
- snoring started, which became 'gross'
- ski gloves would no longer fit his hands
- feet became broader and thicker, and shoe size increased
- chest became so enlarged that people thought he was a weight-lifter, and the sternum became very pronounced

- eyes appeared sunken as face, eyebrows, lips and nose enlarged
- speech changed with slurring of words because the tongue would 'no longer fit my mouth cavity—it was larger than my bite'
- lower jaw moved forward and 'my bite was faulty'
- there was a tendency to persistent colds and influenza
- skin became very sweaty—'I was hot and clammy to touch'
- thirst became excessive
- urine was a dark colour and had a pungent smell
- body hair and 'beard' became thinner
- sex drive reduced but 'performance was normal'
- weight gain was 18 kg but no fat, all 'bulk and muscle'.

Two years previously Mike developed severe lower back pain and visited a chiropractor who felt that he had acromegaly and should report to his family doctor. Amazingly, his doctor dismissed this diagnosis and did not in fact consider the diagnosis during several other visits. Eventually, the doctor did consider it and ordered scans, which detected a very large pituitary tumour.

Outcome
Mike had surgical removal of his pituitary tumour followed by bromocriptine medication. He feels considerably better, but there has been only minimal reversal of his appearance.

The 'elephant man' feeling
The biggest disappointment to Mike was the attitude of his specialist attendants in hospital. He said: 'I felt like a plate of meat—not a person. I really felt like the elephant man. The doctor would come into my hospital room with his entourage and, without asking permission, say with great glee, "Look at this classic case of acromegaly—look at his chest, feel his clammy skin, look at his feet" and so on. There were no explanations about the cause of the tumour or follow-up instructions, and I'm a university graduate'.

DISCUSSION AND LESSONS LEARNED

- Endocrine disorders can develop slowly and subtly under our eyes and the diagnosis can be overlooked, especially in the early stages. The GP has to be sufficiently disciplined to stand back and take a fresh look at the seemingly 'forever complaining' patient.
- It is foolhardy not to take discreet notice of suggestions by patients, family, paramedical or other health professionals about the possible diagnosis. It is wise to follow up this possibility. There may be the threat of litigation if a correct suggestion is not taken seriously.
- The importance of careful explanations about cause, effect and expected outcomes is highlighted here. Patients need and deserve proper education about their diseases as part of the contract they have with their doctors. This was neglected badly with Mike.
- Patients do not appreciate being treated as 'museum pieces'. Their dignity and self-esteem have suffered enough without being stressed by the high-handed and unprofessional conduct of some of our colleagues in hospitals.

A real headache

Mr JT is a 44-year-old tradesman who had been very fit and rarely attended any doctor. He presented to me complaining of an occipital headache. A full neurological examination was normal. His blood pressure was 120/80. I considered that a viral headache was the most likely cause and treated him with simple analgesia and rest.

The next night I was called to visit him as he had developed a severe pounding headache while straining on the toilet. Neurological examination was again normal, but his blood pressure was elevated at 210/80. He was referred to a major public hospital for further assessment.

When I saw him the next day he had undergone a CT scan of his brain, which had proved normal.

Three days later I was called to see him as he had once again developed a severe headache associated with vomiting. Due to the persistence of his headache he was referred back to the public hospital for further assessment. He returned home following a lumbar puncture, which proved normal.

My fourth visit revealed him to have a slight headache and his blood pressure was still elevated at 150/100. Due to the persistence of his hypertension I decided to commence him on felodipine 5 mg daily and order blood urea and electrolytes, which were normal.

JT's blood pressure was well controlled on the felodipine, but I remained suspicious that an undiscovered cause prompted his sudden presentation. I undertook a series of 24-hour urinary catecholamines, especially as he complained of recent occasional palpitations and sweating. To my surprise the series of three 24-hour urinary catch catecholamines strongly suggested the possibility of a phaeochromocytoma (see table below).

RESULTS OF URINARY CATECHOLAMINES

24-hour hydroxymethoxy mandelic acid (HMMA) 430 μmol/day (N:7–24)

	Adrenaline	Dopamine	Noradrenaline
Normal	(90 mmol/dL)	(400–3400 mmol/dL)	(50–650 mmol/dL)
Specimen 1	227	11 812	10 743
Specimen 2	155	11 516	10 927
Specimen 3	154	10 059	9065

Because of these results I ordered a CT scan of his abdomen. This revealed a right-sided adrenal tumour diagnosed as a phaeochromocytoma, which measured about 5 cm in diameter, and had a zone of necrosis laterally (Figure 4.3).

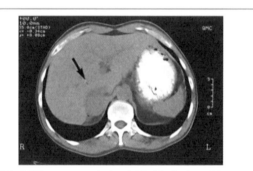

Fig. 4.3 A CT scan revealed a right-sided adrenal tumour

Back in hospital, he underwent a right adrenalectomy under cover with α and β blockage. At operation the right adrenal was found to have been replaced by an encapsulated soft, partly yellow, partly brown mass. There was no evidence of metastatic spread. He made a good recovery and his blood pressure remains normal.

DISCUSSION AND LESSONS LEARNED

- This experience has reinforced the need to be ever vigilant in general practice for possible extraordinary causes of run-of-the-mill problems.
- I have also learnt more about an unusual cause of hypertension, phaeochromocytomas being a rare cause of hypertension occurring in approximately 0.1 per cent of the hypertensive population. For more information, see E M Meumann (Medical free text, 2008).
- The clinical presentation is so variable that phaeochromocytoma has been termed 'the great masquerader' by many endocrinologists.
- Phaeochromocytomas are most common in young to mid-adult life, and patients present most commonly with hypertension. Another presenting symptom complex is a so-called 'crisis', where the patient presents with headache, palpitations, profuse sweating and apprehension. These crises can last from minutes to hours and can occur at varying intervals.
- One of the saddest medico-legal cases I have seen involved the death of a 27-year-old patient following the delivery of her first child. The patient was hypertensive and complained of palpitations post delivery. She was treated with an IV beta blocker and died soon afterwards. Post-mortem revealed a phaeochromocytoma. The patient had a long history of palpitations and 'anxiety attacks'. She had been referred to a cardiologist one year before her death. The cardiologist performed an electrophysiological study but was unable to induce a tachycardia. The patient was referred back to her GP with a diagnosis of anxiety.

Sinister, deadly and not to be missed

Chapter 5

Neisseria meningitidis—modern day 'black death'

The following is a medico-legal case where I was requested to write a report and one of many where I experienced that gut-wrenching feeling of 'there but for the Grace of God go I'.

'Sarah', aged 3 years, attended a general practice one evening because she was unwell, lethargic, febrile, refused to eat and had developed a fine macular rash on her trunk. The examining practitioner noted that she was lying quietly, looked pale and had the pink rash on her chest and back. The only recorded vital sign was a temperature of 38.5 °C (*otic*).

A diagnosis of the viral infection, roseola infantum, was made, paracetamol prescribed, and the parents were advised to return or contact him if her condition deteriorated. Sarah did deteriorate with drowsiness, floppiness, cold extremities, breathing difficulty and a change in the rash to 'black'. Her parents took her to the nearest major hospital, where she was admitted with meningococcal septicaemia. After a lengthy stay she did survive but had to have partial amputations of both arms because of severe ischaemia.

There are many reported cases of children and adults deteriorating and dying with or without prior consultation. The court proceedings were prolonged and harrowing for all concerned. The judge was particularly critical of the GP for failing to record all the vital signs in the history—temperature, pulse rate, blood pressure and respiratory rate.

DISCUSSION AND LESSONS LEARNED

- Acute life-threatening infections such as bacterial meningitis or septicaemia do worry us to distraction and so we should be highly suspicious of these conditions in the sick child and refer if in doubt.
- If we diagnose such a deadly infection and time reaching an emergency centre is a factor it is appropriate to give intravenous benzyl penicillin or cephalosporin (preferable if available).
- The vasculitis of meningococcal septicaemia can start as a mild maculopapular rash that resembles a mild viral exanthema prior to the classic haemorrhagic rash.
- Useful early signs include the following: an inactive disinterested child, cold skin particularly of the extremities, decreased capillary return, increased work of breathing and reduced mental state.

Stress, angina, smokes, Viagra and *angor animi*

Chuck was a 55-year-old American general practitioner who was our house guest for a few days. Arriving in Australia for a holiday, he commenced his journey to Melbourne from Cairns in a rented motor home. When he arrived, he said that the long trip on unfamiliar roads was so stressful that he had resorted to chain smoking. He said that he had a history of angina pectoris and was taking glyceryl trinitrate by pump spray for any chest pain. He retired saying that he felt more relaxed and was looking forward to a good night's sleep.

At midnight we heard a commotion in the upstairs bathroom where we found a deathly pale, vomiting and sweating Chuck with chest pain and classic *angor animi*. He was terrified and using his glyceryl trinitrate spray indiscriminately.

It was obvious that he had suffered a myocardial infarction and looked as though cardiac arrest was imminent. We rang for the MICA ambulance and gave him soluble aspirin. The ambulance arrived in about 10 minutes and performed an ECG which showed an anterior infarction and then transported him to the nearby major hospital. His wife informed me that he had taken Viagra and was having sex when the pain struck.

When he arrived at the hospital emergency department after a fast 15-minute trip he had a cardiac arrest and was successfully resuscitated with defibrillation. He was then whisked off to the coronary catheter laboratory where he had a stent placed in the left anterior descending artery. When we visited him nine hours later he looked well, as though nothing dramatic had eventuated during the night.

DISCUSSION AND LESSONS LEARNED

- Chuck had several coronary risk factors and as a doctor should have known better than to smoke, take Viagra and then suck glyceryl trinitrate constantly.
- The importance of time in making a diagnosis, getting a coronary care ambulance, emergency expertise and definitive intervention with coronary angiography and percutaneous intervention (or CABGs) was obvious.
- Chuck could not believe his good fortune especially with the relatively modest size of the bills for the services provided. A spectacular bowl of flowers and fruit have arrived at the hospital emergency department and at our home on the anniversary of his heart attack for the past five years.

Guess what?

Case 1

'Will you come down to the hospital to see yet another football player? He doesn't look too good. Probably has broken ribs and pneumothorax.'

'Typical Saturday afternoon,' I thought as I went to see Robert S, aged 22. Robert was holding a painful precordium and looking pale and sweaty. 'Did you get a heavy knock?' 'No, not really.' His chest was normal on clinical examination. 'If he was older I'd think it was myocardial infarction,' I thought just before he moaned loudly and then collapsed.

Resuscitation, despite optimal facilities, was unsuccessful. Autopsy showed acute myocardial infarction (AMI).

Case 2

Lila J, aged 62, was the local Methodist minister's wife, a truly beautiful person who attended me for hypertension. One evening I was called to her home because I was told: 'Mum is complaining of a funny constricting feeling in her throat and is having trouble breathing. We've had fish for tea and we think she must be allergic to it'.

I hurried to treat the acute allergic problem, only to find a very pale and anxious-looking lady who said, 'My throat is tight and closing up'. As I nervously felt a slow and irregular pulse, she had a cardiac arrest.

To the horror of the onlooking loved ones, I commenced cardiopulmonary resuscitation and asked one of the relatives to bring in my portable defibrillator. This was successful initially but she died some time later in hospital.

Case 3

Alan P, aged 49, is a mountain of a man who uses jackhammers each day as he drills through concrete. He presented one afternoon looking quite well but claiming, 'This work is catching up with me—I've had terribly aching arms all day'. Further questioning revealed that he had the pain in both forearms for five hours and then reluctantly came in when he felt 'lightheaded and peculiar'. I could find nothing abnormal on examination but intuitively took blood for cardiac enzymes and performed an ECG—another AMI.

Case 4

Mary B, a 41-year-old woman, presented with the sudden onset of severe pain in the interscapular area of her back. However, I could find no abnormality on examination of her thoracic spine. My provisional diagnosis included a pathological fracture in an osteoporotic vertebra, but a routine ECG provided the answer to the unusual presentation—AMI and not a twinge of discomfort in the anterior chest.

Case 5

I was called to see Sarah C, a 72-year-old diabetic, at 3 am because of the sudden onset of dyspnoea. 'An easy one,' I thought as I sped to the farmhouse. 'Morphine, frusemide and oxygen will fix her acute pulmonary oedema in no time. Love treating them.' Well, that treatment did not make any impression on her distress (anxiety, sweating, dyspnoea). Unfortunately, she died in hospital from the complications of her AMI. Never a complaint of chest pain—a truly silent AMI that precipitated acute cardiac failure.

Case 6

A first-aid person rang me one afternoon to say that 78-year-old Minnie P had been run over by a car in the main street of the town. 'She's in bad shape— multiple fractures, ribs and left humerus at least.'

My first sighting in the emergency department was a 'shocked' elderly lady with abrasions who was moaning with pain. She pointed to her sternum, precordium and left arm. There was no clinical evidence of fractures. I quickly organised an ECG, which confirmed AMI. Minnie died two hours later. The attending policeman said, 'The driver has been let off the hook. He was emphatic that she suddenly fell onto the road and then under the car as she was crossing it in front of him'.

Case 7

Phyllis M, aged 62, a close relative of the author, requested another opinion about severe epigastric pains and 'indigestion' diagnosed as a peptic ulcer but unrelieved by antacids and H_2 antagonists. It was a real brain teaser, but her obvious pallor and discomfort prompted an ECG, which confirmed a recent AMI.

DISCUSSION AND LESSONS LEARNED

- Acute coronary syndromes and coronary artery disease in general are common and can be easily missed, especially if presentation is atypical (an estimated 10–30 per cent of patients with AMI have an 'atypical presentation'), as highlighted in these case histories.

- It is vital to make an early diagnosis of these cases and transfer patients to a specialist coronary care unit. Statistics show that most deaths occur in the first one to two hours, and that chances of survival are improved significantly in these special units and with the attendance of special intensive-care ambulances. Ideally we prefer to have these patients admitted to a coronary intervention unit within 60–90 minutes of the onset of pain.

- It appears to be easier to overlook an acute coronary syndrome (AMI) in the context of a busy surgery, especially as so many causes of chest pain are not, as expected, due to coronary insufficiency.

- The advent of more sensitive cardiac enzyme markers such as the troponins has improved our diagnostic rate.

- Age appears to be no barrier to diagnosis; approximately 2–6 per cent of AMIs occur in patients younger than 40 years, a group often considered to be too young to have an AMI.

- Smoking, hyperlipidaemia, diabetes mellitus and hypertension are obviously common associations in these patients. I refer to these as 'the Four Horsemen of the Apocalypse'.

- In patients who present with 'atypical' chest pain or other symptoms that could be cardiac in origin, GPs need to maintain a high index of suspicion for acute coronary syndrome, particularly in those patients with known cardiac risk factors.

- Failure to diagnose AMI is a common cause of claims and complaints against GPs. The most common incorrect diagnoses made by GPs are gastrointestinal problems and musculoskeletal pain, such as costochondritis.

- An emerging area of medico-legal risk for GPs is an allegation of failure to appropriately diagnose or manage cardiac risk factors, resulting in AMI.

Lethal family histories

Case 1

Betty R was a 68-year-old ex-nurse living in retirement in a pleasant rural area when she presented for a general check-up. She claimed to be in good health but had been bothered slightly by 'sluggish bowels' and vague abdominal discomfort for the past year or so. She had a long history of mild hypertension for which she was taking low-dose beta blockers. She was a very matter-of-fact 'now you see her, now you don't' type of person who conveyed the impression that she felt that she was bothering her doctor and wanted to get on her way with her script.

During this particular consultation I sensed that she was ready for some dialogue and perhaps reassurance. Fortunately, I asked that marvellous question, 'Do you have any particular concerns about your health?'

'Yes' she said, reflectively yet urgently. 'I am the only surviving member of my family. They all seemed to die mysteriously around the age of 70. I remember that my father died quite suddenly. He was in great pain and went very pale. No one seems to know what he died from—it was very strange, no postmortem was done. They thought it was a heart attack. My sister, who lived alone, was found dead in bed although she had been quite well the previous day. She had cancer of the breast, but her death at 65 years was sooner than expected.

'The death of my brother at 69 about six years ago really upset me. He was in the country and developed severe pains in the back and stomach. He was rushed to a city hospital but was dead on arrival. I don't know what he died from.'

Diagnosis

This challenging history fascinated me and obviously caused Betty considerable anxiety. Her brother's history started me thinking about ruptured aneurysms of the abdominal aorta, and knowing the familial history of such lesions I directed my physical examination carefully towards the abdomen.

Abdominal palpation revealed the characteristic pulsatile mass of an abdominal aneurysm, which I estimated at about 50 to 60 mm.

Betty had been unaware of the presence of an abdominal mass, but said she felt that something had been wrong with her stomach because it 'felt tender and uncomfortable at times'.

I reassured her that we had discovered the probable cause of the family malady and that her outlook was fine. I organised an ultrasound examination, a referral to a vascular surgeon and wrote to Flinders Medical Centre for details about the possible cause of death of her brother.

Outcome

Ultrasound examination showed an aneurysm about 60 mm in diameter. I eventually found out that her brother had died from a ruptured aneurysm of his abdominal aorta.

Betty underwent surgical repair three weeks later. The surgeon was alarmed to find 'a paper-thin wall to the diseased vessel' and one can only speculate on how inevitable a rupture would be. Despite the setback of a pulmonary embolus, Betty is now fit and well and ponders over her good fortune, but she worries about her seven children now entering middle age.

Case 2

Eric P was a fit 59-year-old bus driver who presented to me for a check-up and discussion about his family history. His father had died suddenly aged 62 from a 'heart attack', and a brother had also died suddenly at 60 from a 'heart attack' and yet another surviving brother who was a smoker suffered a 'heart attack' at 56 years. A common feature was the suddenness of the myocardial infarction without any preceding angina or other ill health.

Eric had been so aware of this poor family history that he had been meticulous with his health and lifestyle. He kept fit and trim, followed a strict diet, did not smoke or drink and practised relaxation.

Physical examination, chest X-ray and an ECG revealed no abnormalities. In particular, his cardiac function and blood pressure were normal. I organised a stress ECG test that provoked some chest discomfort typical of angina at high stress. Ischaemic changes were noted on the stress ECG.

I decided to refer him to a cardiologist for further evaluation. About 10 days later while awaiting his appointment (due in four days' time) he suddenly collapsed. He was dead on arrival at the hospital.

DISCUSSION AND LESSONS LEARNED

- We ignore a significant family history at our patients' (and our own) peril. These case histories reinforce the importance of taking and recording the family history of all our patients.
- Aneurysms of the abdominal aorta have a familial tendency and where relevant it is wise to screen relatives for this abnormality. The investigations of choice are ultrasound and computerised tomography with the latter providing better imaging.
- By definition, an aneurysm of the abdominal aorta is one that is greater than 30 mm in diameter; greater than 50 mm represents significant enlargement and the arbitrary reference point to consider surgery; and greater than 60 mm represents danger.
- Eric's untimely death was a lesson. The cardiologist felt that his anxiety provoked a fatal arrhythmia and that in hindsight prescribing beta blockers straight after his stress ECG could have helped. It is possible that coronary angiography and bypass may have been life saving.
- The cardiologist also stressed the importance of a phone call from the onset so that he was aware of the patient and the problem and could offer immediate advice.

The wrong pipeline

It was one of those occasions in the life of an overworked country doctor when the impending arrival of the locum produced visions of relaxation in a subtropical resort. The ringing of the phone jolted me back to reality. An anxious farmer informed me that his wife had suddenly developed an agonising pain in the middle of her back, which had persisted for an hour.

The inevitable thoughts sped through my mind as he spoke: 'Another back problem. Surely it will subside. The locum can handle it. Well, it sounds unusual—rather like the old dowagers who suddenly collapse their osteoporotic vertebrae. Faye is young, trim and healthy—what could it be? What if it's a dissecting aneurysm? Perhaps I should see her immediately'.

I saw an agitated Faye (42 years old and previously healthy) at the hospital 20 minutes later and found that she still had pain between the shoulder blades at the T4–T5 level. There was no anterior chest pain, nausea, dyspnoea or any other symptom. On examination there was absolutely nothing abnormal: no pallor, no inequality of the pulses and no spinal tenderness. The hypotheses continued to flow: 'Could she have an acute disc prolapse? They are epidemic here in the bush. What about myocardial infarction? That is really a master of disguise and I saw a similar case five years ago. Time for an ECG'.

The locum arrived as I was performing the ECG in Faye's hospital room and he confirmed my assessment of a normal tracing. We discussed the differential diagnosis and the management plan, which included an intramuscular injection of morphine, hospitalisation and an X-ray of her thoracic spine.

Diagnosis

The pain soon settled and, apart from general weakness, Faye was quite well until two days later when she suddenly developed twitching of the right side of her face, dysphasia, blurred vision and hemianaesthesia of her right side. This dramatic two-hour long episode provoked a phone call to a neurologist who arranged her admission to a city hospital. Several investigations including a skull X-ray, electroencephalogram (EEG) and a brain scan were performed, and all were negative. A diagnosis of anxiety and depression was attached to the patient who was discharged with a 'magic remedy'—amitriptyline.

Faye consulted me on the first day after my holidays, and she complained of extreme fatigue and light headedness. She appeared listless and pale, but the only abnormalities on physical examination were an irregular pulse and crepitations at both lung bases.

Further investigations

A repeat ECG showed evidence of an anterior myocardial infarction with ventricular ectopic beats. A chest X-ray and haemoglobin estimation were normal.

She had had a myocardial infarct after all. The cerebral ischaemic episode was caused probably by an embolus from a left ventricular thrombosis associated with a transmural infarct. (Using serial two-dimensional echocardiography, Asinger and his co-workers (1981) have demonstrated that left ventricular thrombus can develop 1 to 11 days after an acute transmural anterior infarct.)

The subsequent deterioration in her health with a cardiac arrhythmia (ventricular ectopic beats) and mild congestive cardiac failure was probably related to the tricyclic antidepressant.

DISCUSSION AND LESSONS LEARNED

- A potentially lethal myocardial infarction can present in many ways and the diagnosis can be missed. Masquerades include back pain, epigastric pain, precordial pain, jaw pain, arm pain and 'heartburn'. Infarction may be even painless (up to 20 per cent of cases). Women, diabetics and older patients are more likely to present without chest pain, but have symptoms of dyspnoea, weakness, nausea and vomiting, palpitations or syncope.
- A relatively young, fit person is certainly not immune to myocardial infarction. It is not uncommon among people in their twenties and it has been recorded in fit, young athletes.
- A negative ECG taken in the early stages does not exclude a myocardial infarct. It may take up to six hours before the classic initial ECG abnormalities appear. Occasionally an infarct, invariably subendocardial, will not produce an ECG change at any stage. We should have repeated the ECG in this patient although her history was not typical. A follow-up with serial cardiac enzymes was imperative and this was omitted.
- One of the highlights of this case was the inappropriate referral but one should not be too critical of the specialist. In this age of specialisation it is

- often very difficult for specialists to think laterally, and thus it exposes the increasing responsibility and importance of the general practitioner to screen patients and direct them along the right 'pipeline' to the appropriate specialist.
- It is shattering for patients who have a genuine organic problem to be informed that their malady is caused by 'nerves'. Unfortunately, we often resort to inappropriate counselling, perhaps to mask our ignorance.
- Tricyclic antidepressants can be very dangerous in the early convalescent phase of an acute myocardial infarction (AMI). The patient improved dramatically when they were ceased. In fact, the manufacturers list this period as a contraindication to their use.

'I think she's carked it'

Anne W was the 32-year-old kindergarten teacher of our children and also a personal friend. At 5 am on Easter Saturday I received an urgent call from her shaken husband to come to see her at their country school residence. Upon arrival some 20 minutes later, I found the glamorous Anne sitting up in bed saying, 'I don't know what all the panic is about—I feel fine now'. Her husband said, 'Anne woke me calling out with severe stomach pain. She looked pale and dreadful—frightening'. Anne said that the pain in her lower abdomen lasted only 10 to 15 minutes. 'I've been having trouble with my periods—bleeding when it shouldn't—I think I need a change of the pill. I've made an appointment to see you on Monday.'

After palpating a normal-feeling abdomen I was about to perform a pelvic examination, but the body language in that bedroom said, 'Don't touch—I'm comfortable—Don't embarrass all of us with an internal'. So 'chicken doctor' flew back home.

Diagnosis and outcome

On Easter Sunday I was called out of church. It was Anne. 'Flat as a tack,' said her neighbour, 'I think she's carked it. You'd better come quick.' 'Bloody ectopic,' I thought as I sped off. 'I dismissed it yesterday. She's on the pill. Why didn't I do a pelvic examination?'

I arrived to find a semi-comatose woman, of a similar colour to the sheets in which she lay, looking quite moribund. A quick cut down onto the cephalic vein and then intravenous Hartmann's solution followed by Haemaccel brought an encouragingly rapid response with her blood pressure rising from 50/30 to 90/50. I sent her husband with a sample of blood for typing and cross-matching on the long trip to the base hospital to get blood, and then I transferred her to our bush nursing hospital. At surgery her abdomen was full of blood from the ruptured ectopic pregnancy. Once the bleeding was arrested and the transfusion commenced, the drama subsided.

During the ward round the following morning the glamorous Anne sat up in bed with make-up and bedwear fit for a film star. 'Someone's saved my life. I feel fine now,' she said. And all without a vaginal examination, I mused.

DISCUSSION AND LESSONS LEARNED

- The ectopic pregnancy is potentially lethal and demands the utmost respect. My old gynaecology teacher would drum it into us: 'Think ectopic—be ectopic-minded—think ectopic'. Sometimes we do not think it, and sometimes we think it but dismiss it, when it is there—lurking.
- Treating friends is very difficult, especially in circumstances such as Anne's. Although rectal and vaginal examinations can be uncomfortable to all involved parties the 'bullet has to be bitten', for it gets back to the old medical aphorism: 'If you don't put your finger in it, you'll put your foot in it'.
- Ectopic pregnancies can occur in the presence of contraception (the pill, intrauterine devices and barrier methods) and patients may give a normal menstrual history.
- The golden rule should be: 'If a woman of child-bearing age presents with the sudden onset of lower abdominal pain, she has an ectopic pregnancy until proved otherwise'.

IUDs and ectopic pregnancy

Sue T, a 27-year-old mother of two, consulted me 24 hours before admission to hospital for the biopsy of a breast lump detected three weeks previously.

She described 19 days of painless vaginal bleeding beginning with the previous menstrual period. She interpreted this as a prolonged period related to the stress of the pending breast surgery.

Twelve months ago I had inserted a Copper 7 intrauterine contraceptive device (IUD), which had proved very satisfactory apart from an occasional heavy period. She had not missed a period. I informed her that the persistent bleeding was probably due to the IUD, which should be removed. I could not remove it in the surgery because I could not locate the string.

I arranged that the surgeon would remove the IUD and perform a dilatation and curettage (D and C) during the breast biopsy procedure. He reported that the uterus seemed slightly enlarged but that no masses were palpable. She returned to me 10 days later complaining of lower abdominal pain for seven days, worse on defecation and micturition, persistent minimal vaginal bleeding and dyspareunia. Pelvic examination revealed a slight enlargement of the uterus and tenderness in the left fornix and Pouch of Douglas.

I arranged an appointment with a gynaecologist the following day, but her husband phoned me two hours later to say that the pain was now intense and that she had virtually 'collapsed'. She was admitted to hospital immediately and the gynaecologist performed a laparoscopy, which confirmed an ectopic pregnancy of about six weeks' gestation in the left fallopian tube. Salpingectomy was then performed.

DISCUSSION AND LESSONS LEARNED

- **The diagnosis** The ectopic pregnancy can be a real masquerade in general practice and we should always be 'ectopic-minded' with women of child-bearing age who have unusual menstrual bleeding or lower abdominal pain. Current contraceptive use or even sterilisation should not deter one from considering this possibility; not keeping the diagnosis in mind can contribute to an embarrassing tragedy.
- **The missed period** The absence of amenorrhoea can be a trap in failing to diagnose pregnancy. Many ectopic pregnancies have a history of regular periods albeit altered in nature.

- **The IUD** Pregnancy should be suspected in any patient with an IUD who has prolonged or heavy bleeding. Ectopic pregnancy should be suspected in a patient with vaginal bleeding, an enlarged uterus and an IUD, especially if pain is present. Remove the IUD if possible as soon as pregnancy is confirmed.
- **The dilatation and curettage** There is a tendency to regard early ectopic pregnancies as incomplete abortions. Examining the patient under anaesthesia and performing a dilatation and curettage can lull one into a false sense of security that the problem has been dealt with definitively.
- Once ectopic pregnancy is diagnosed, surgical intervention, which carries risks of haemorrhage and subsequent hysterectomy, may not be necessary. Maternal intramuscular methotrexate is first-line treatment.

Unravelling problematic asthma

Case 1

One evening I was called to our local hospital to an emergency. When I arrived I found a comatose and cyanosed 14-year-old lad who was beyond resuscitation. I recognised him as an asthmatic patient whom I had not seen for some time. According to his distressed mother, his asthma had been getting worse recently and had culminated in this fatal attack.

The mother explained that the family were unhappy about him inhaling 'cortisone' and drugs that make the heart race, and they sought the help of a naturopath who claimed that he could cure asthma. The patient then stopped his prescribed medication and underwent 'herb and vitamin therapy' as well as spinal manipulation. This sad occasion was not the time to pass comment about such treatment.

Case 2

Dennis W, aged 22, attended one of my adult asthma education groups that are open to the public. He said that he had been self-medicating with salbutamol inhalers all his life.

I lent him a peak flow meter to accurately assess his respiratory function. The readings were unacceptable to both of us. He agreed to commence inhaled corticosteroids, and the improvements in his asthma (Figure 5.1), general health and morale were amazing.

Case 3

Margaret M, aged 67, had late-onset asthma that showed unacceptable control. In fact the medication seemed to make little difference. I organised peak flow readings and studied her inhaler technique. The latter was faulty. We could not seem to correct her technique and so we introduced a spacer.

The change in her asthmatic control was dramatic and she has achieved a greatly improved quality of life.

DISCUSSION AND LESSONS LEARNED

- Asthma is a deadly condition with an unacceptable mortality rate. The importance of better understanding of patient's control and management, through the doctor spending more time in education or through an adult education course, has been obvious through my many experiences conducting such courses.
- Poor patient delivery technique is an important cause of inadequate control, insufficient compliance and severe, perhaps fatal, attacks.
- Apart from pumps and nebulisers, there have been three outstanding advances in the modern management of bronchial asthma:
  - the use of spirometry and the mini peak flow meter
  - the use of spacers attached to inhalers/puffers
  - the realisation that asthma is an inflammatory disease and inhaled corticosteroids or sodium cromoglycate is appropriate first- or second-line treatment for persistent asthma.
- Self-medication is unacceptable—the patient requires regular monitoring. In particular alternative non-scientific therapies claiming cure should be discouraged or at least carefully evaluated.

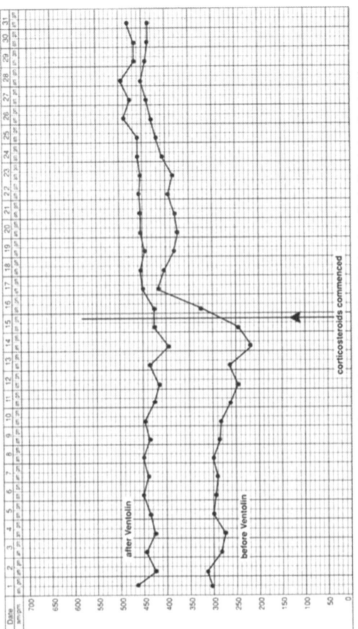

Fig. 5.1 Dennis W: graph of morning peak flows (before and after Ventolin) showing effect of inhaled corticosteroids

Living with one's mistakes

Kate M, the 35-year-old wife of a teacher, made a striking impression when she first consulted me in my country practice. A beautiful person with a vivacious personality, she presented for a prescription for a tranquilliser because of an 'anxiety state'. When the consultation appeared terminated she casually mentioned: 'Perhaps you should check my breasts. I had them checked a month ago by my previous doctor who said they were healthy but required "watching"'. A rather hurried examination revealed large heavy breasts with diffuse fibroadenotic thickening, the left breast lumpier than the right. Pinning excessive faith on the judgement of her previous practitioner, I concluded that they seemed okay but should be reviewed in six months. Breast self-examination was discussed. No imaging was available then.

Three months later Kate presented with a trivial complaint and again said: 'Perhaps you should check my breasts before I go'. As I looked at the breasts I suddenly felt nauseated and tremulous as I could see skin dimpling over the left breast. A hard mass was tethered to the skin.

Three days later the surgeon phoned to confidently prognosticate: 'It went well—we got all of the tumour—there were no involved nodes— stage 1—no further treatment will be necessary'. This news helped alleviate my guilt and embarrassment as I relayed the information to her husband who had posed the obvious question: 'How come you guys didn't pick this up beforehand?'

Four months later Kate presented with a small hard lump in the scar and the 'nightmare' started. Carcinoma! Radiotherapy—another lump—cytotoxic therapy—extreme nausea, syncopal attacks, *alopecia totalis*—corticosteroid therapy—Cushingoid features—depression—multiple somatic complaints. She grew grotesque while deteriorating medically, and I wished that the cytotoxic torture had never started. I felt bad—really bad. My guilt became sublimated into zealous caring, manifested in many impromptu home visits.

On one occasion she complained of an aching right thigh. Examination was quite normal so I reassured her it was probably 'muscular' and nothing to worry about. Two days later she was found lying on the kitchen floor with a fractured femur caused by a pathological fracture through a metastatic deposit in the femoral shaft.

Several days later I was called urgently to the hospital where she was convalescing from the insertion of a Küntscher nail by an orthopaedic surgeon. Kate was dead, less than 12 months after the initial consultation. She had called for a bed pan as a pulmonary embolus swiftly and kindly terminated the medical 'merry-go-round'.

DISCUSSION AND LESSONS LEARNED

- Lumpy fibroadenotic breasts and breast lumps in general can be difficult problems for the 'front line' doctor. There is no place for rushed examinations or playing a waiting game for the breast tissue to declare itself. Follow Cancer Australia's *The investigation of a new breast symptom—a guide for General Practitioners* (2017), which recommends a triple-test approach to diagnosis. Ensure follow-up of patients with breast symptoms and/or signs to resolution.
- We should be more sensitive to patients' anxieties and sense that they wish to draw attention to something such as an unusual lump, despite presenting with some other complaint.
- Do not discount the possibility of breast cancer because of a patient's young age—low risk does not mean no risk.
- We should pay careful attention to any unusual symptoms and signs in patients who have a known primary carcinoma, albeit excised many years previously.
- Living with our mistakes can be a great teacher and very humbling. As one wise teacher used to say: 'The only real mistake is the one from which we learn nothing'.

Sidetracked

Mrs F, aged 53, presented with a four-week history of altered bowel habit, having diarrhoea and unsatisfied defecation. Her symptoms had begun about two weeks after a very pleasant four-week trip to South-East Asia. She felt quite well and had a normal appetite. There were minimal abdominal cramps and her stool was abnormal; on one occasion she had observed blood and mucus.

A full blood examination, microscopy and culture of the stools ordered at this visit revealed an eosinophilia, an ESR of 45 and also cysts of the parasite *Giardia lamblia* in the stool. The patient was given a course of metronidazole.

On review one week later her bowel actions were improved. A repeat course of metronidazole was prescribed and a full blood examination was performed two weeks later. This revealed no eosinophilia, and ESR was 15. She was told to return in four weeks if her bowel actions were not completely normal. She did, complaining of further symptoms—the passage of mucus with flatus and the occasional sensation of prolapse of the bowel on defecation.

Diagnosis

A rectal examination revealed a mass with a heaped margin at the tip of the gloved finger. Sigmoidoscopy confirmed a large annular ulcerated mass at 9 cm, which was bleeding. Biopsy demonstrated adenocarcinoma and an anterior resection was performed. Incidentally, the patient had a strong family history of carcinoma of the bowel.

DISCUSSION AND LESSONS LEARNED

- The first mistake was not to perform a complete physical examination. The old medical aphorism: 'If you don't put your finger in it, you'll put your foot in it' is vividly demonstrated with this patient.
- The establishment of one diagnosis does not preclude the possibility of another. Although the evidence favouring *Giardia* was convincing, the persistence of symptoms indicating carcinoma was not disregarded.

Giardiasis is a relatively common infestation that is frequently overlooked. However, the cardinal feature of this infection is persistent watery diarrhoea.

- A significant history can never be lightly dismissed.

Keeping a stiff upper lip

The patient, a very sprightly 79-year-old woman, rang on a Monday morning complaining of a sore throat and asked for a home visit. She usually walked the kilometre from her home to the surgery for checks on her blood pressure and asthma status and so I knew she was 'genuine'.

When I was at the bedside, she complained of pain in the mouth and on the left side of the face. On examination she looked unwell and the left parotid duct orifice was swollen and oozing saliva. The provisional diagnosis was parotid duct calculus with superimposed infection, and appropriate treatment was commenced. Unfortunately, during the afternoon she became unsteady on her feet and fell twice, hurting her neck.

On review the next day she was a little worse; examination of the buccal cavity was limited because she found it difficult to open her mouth fully. Her neck was tender with considerable muscle spasm and she complained of cramps in her left leg. It was considered wise to admit her to hospital for further investigation and nursing care because she lived alone.

The specialist surgical opinion sought in the hospital agreed with the likelihood of a parotid duct calculus, but full blood examination and X-ray of the parotid region were normal. The diagnosis first occurred to me that afternoon, and after rejecting it a dozen times in my mind I broached the possibility, almost self-deprecatingly, to the surgeon who felt it was possible, albeit rare.

Diagnosis and outcome

The charge nurse rang early the next morning to say that the patient was breathless—could I come to see her? On examination she was perspiring profusely and was having a mild to moderate attack of asthma. When on my suggestion she attempted to use her bronchodilator inhaler she could barely open her mouth wide enough to insert the mouthpiece.

Becoming bolder (after reading the relevant chapter in *Harrison's Principles of Internal Medicine*) and after further consultation and examination by a specialist physician—who felt the diagnosis was possible but uncertain—she was transferred to the infectious diseases hospital. Later that night she experienced further and more severe tetanic spasms and was intubated.

Despite suffering a myocardial infarction in the ensuing weeks, she survived her brush with tetanus and, after three months in hospital, was almost back to her former sprightly self.

DISCUSSION AND LESSONS LEARNED

- I was always taught that an uncommon presentation of a common illness was more frequent than a common presentation of an uncommon illness. Therefore, think of common things first. However, that does not mean that you can forget rare diseases.
- Tetanus exists and is a potentially lethal disease. A total of 10 to 20 per cent of patients with tetanus have no identifiable wound of entry (Isselbacher et al., 1991).
- Tetanus is a preventable disease; encourage immunisation in all patients at routine visits.
- Do not be frightened to back your medical intuition; it is an important part of the diagnostic process.

A snake in the grass

It was a balmy April afternoon and outside a thick pall of smoke from the burning bush hung lazily in the autumn sky. Suddenly, the tranquillity was disturbed by the urgent screeching of brakes from a Forests Commission four-wheel drive vehicle at the surgery door. Two brawny foresters burst into the waiting room supporting their stuporose mate by the arms.

'Doc, we thought that you should give Mick 'ere a check-up. He seems to have one hell of a hangover but it's getting worse. He's vomited blood twice and he's staggering all over the place.' These hard-playing boys had seen it all before.

A very drowsy 20-year-old Mick then laboriously explained his problem. The previous evening he had been drinking heavily and playing cards with his mates in their mountain bush shack. This morning he had felt wretched with nausea, tiredness and headache when he started to burn off the low bush in the eucalypt forest. During the lunch break he felt worse: pains in the legs and abdomen, excessive sweating, severe nausea and headache. He received little sympathy from his workmates who berated him for his intolerance of alcohol.

He rested during the afternoon but still felt as if he 'wanted to die'. After he had vomited blood twice and complained of blurred vision, his colleagues dumped him in the Land Rover and headed in my direction.

On examination he was pale, very weak and stuporose. His pulse was 90, with weak volume. BP was 95/60. There was mild abdominal tenderness but no guarding. A neurological examination of the cranial nerves was difficult; no specific abnormalities were detected. There was some voluntary muscular weakness but his reflexes were intact. During the examination he coughed up a moderate quantity of blood-stained mucus.

Diagnosis and outcome

A provisional diagnosis of tiger snake envenomation was made. Mick could not recall having seen any snakes nor remember being bitten, but the undergrowth was waist high and he had felt many scratches and stings from the dry bush as he ran through. Specific examination of the legs revealed the telltale evidence of a snake bite: two small puncture wounds with a slight ooze of unclotted blood halfway up the right leg.

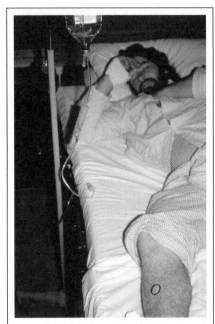

Fig. 5.2 Mick in hospital under treatment for tiger snake envenomation

He was admitted immediately to the local bush nursing hospital (Figure 5.2). We gave him an intravenous infusion of saline, added 25 mg of promethazine and then infused 3000 units of tiger snake antivenene, keeping a syringe with 1 mL of 1:1000 adrenaline nearby.

Mick was very weak and ill for three to four days. During the next six months he battled with a severe depressive illness. His relatives and friends claimed he was a completely different person, complaining of fatigue, multiple somatic complaints and an inability to work. He was weepy and suicidal. Fortunately, his recovery was complete albeit two years later.

DISCUSSION AND LESSONS LEARNED
- Even if the patient does not recall being bitten, always remember the possibility of snake bite in the Australian bush—especially in the case of children or bushworkers.
- Snake bites can occur in late spring, summer, and in autumn when snakes are mating.
- Country practices should always have available an updated supply of snake antivenom.
- Beware of depressive illness after recovery from a severe snake bite.

A female relative with irritable bowel syndrome—or a 'red herring'?

The status of 'doctor' within a family, especially an extended family, brings many requests for help which at least can be a learning experience, especially from the 'cautionary tales' perspective. One such case was that of first cousin 'Mary' who sought advice about a persistent 'irritable bowel syndrome'. The condition had been present for 18 months and she had several visits to at least two doctors in the clinic. She had presented with vague lower abdominal discomfort. She found any pressure from clothing on the abdomen to be tight and uncomfortable. Throughout this period she gradually became flat and unwell and prone to episodes of constipation and diarrhoea. The diagnosis of irritable bowel syndrome seemed logical.

In recent weeks she had become anorexic and noticed weight loss. I was very concerned but did not want to interfere with her management so I suggested that she make an appointment with her GP as soon as possible. She was ordered an ultrasound and tumour markers which suggested carcinoma of the ovary. A laparotomy confirmed the presence of a large tumour causing tethering of pelvic structures. Surgery was eventually performed followed by chemotherapy. Despite a poor prognosis Mary was coping well after three years but, like so many having cytotoxic therapy, remained afflicted with the cold burning feet of peripheral neuropathy.

DISCUSSION AND LESSONS LEARNED

- Carcinoma of the ovary is one of the so-called occult cancers which tends to remain asymptomatic for a long period and then can cause a multitude of whimsical symptoms particularly masquerading as irritable bowel syndrome.
- It is preferable not to become too involved with the medical problems of relatives, including not being perceived as intruding on the management of colleagues. However, it is a privilege to be able to help and advise in a diplomatic, caring way. This applies particularly to one's own children and their children.

Warfarin and INR—a dangerous game

The following potpourri of cases from GP colleagues highlight the fact that warfarin is a major cause of threats to patient safety.

Mr JP, aged 78, presented with a large mass in the left hypochondrium after taking a double dose of warfarin. He was admitted to hospital with a provisional diagnosis of a splenic haemorrhage but was found to have a haematoma of the rectal sheath. He seemed to have little understanding of warfarin action, dosage and monitoring.

Mrs GL, aged 80, who was taking warfarin for atrial fibrillation, was prescribed a non-steroidal anti-inflammatory drug (NSAID) by a specialist for pain management. A rapid rise in her international normalised ratio (INR) followed by haematemesis and melaena from gastric haemorrhage led to a fatal outcome despite multiple transfusions.

Mr IT, aged 80, was discharged from the surgical hospital on warfarin for a pulmonary embolism following treatment for a fractured hip. He then spent 20 weeks in a bush nursing facility and base hospital before going home. When reviewed he was taking warfarin 2 mg bd as directed on the bottle from the original hospital. Both patient and family were confused. His INR was 4.5.

Ms AH, aged 58, who presented with rectal bleeding, was taking warfarin 5 mg daily for atrial fibrillation. Her INR was 11.0. She had spent four weeks interstate and missed her INR-warfarin monitoring by her regular GP. Luckily, she settled without incident.

Mrs ML, aged 57, was admitted to hospital for a transient ischaemic attack and was discharged after warfarin was commenced. The following day she presented with a large haemorrhagic area on her right thigh. It became necrotic and then we battled to treat the ulcer for several months. It was a localised thrombosis apparently related to protein C deficiency and a large loading dose of warfarin.

DISCUSSION AND LESSONS LEARNED

- Problems with warfarin medication are common with the Threats to Australian Patient Safety (TAPS) study reporting a large number of errors (Makeham et al., 2008).

- The elderly and cognitively challenged are particularly vulnerable to errors.
- Patient education on commencing warfarin is an important responsibility of the clinician who initiates therapy, while we as GPs should reinforce messages related to safety and monitoring.
- An excellent strategy is where doctors from pathology laboratories contact both patient and referring doctor about test results, recommended dosage and follow-up.
- We welcome the advent of the clotting factor inhibitors, such as dabigatran, the new generation oral direct anticoagulants, which are more patient friendly and easier to manage, apart from concerns about reversal and overdosage.

Chapter 6

See a doctor, support a lawyer

21 years of iatrogenic abdominal pain

Long ago, during my term as a surgical registrar I was asked to see a rather rugged 65-year-old farmer with chronic intermittent abdominal pain. The problem was puzzling the Resident Medical Officer (RMO), especially as the patient had the 'thick file' syndrome. He was a rather likeable phlegmatic man who seemed to have a genuine problem and was embarrassed by his occasional visits to various doctors and the emergency department. He described the pain, which was located centrally, as colicky, mild to moderate and dull. It was associated with mild abdominal distension, nausea (no vomiting) and constipation with hard, pellet-like stools. Diagnoses that had been suggested were irritable bowel syndrome and/or abdominal adhesions. He said that the painful attacks which simply felt like 'a kick in the guts' would dissipate as quickly as they came. He had a history of a cholecystectomy 21 years previously.

On abdominal examination he had mild central tenderness with rebound tenderness, minor swelling and the suggestion of a firm mass. We did not have sophisticated imaging such as ultrasound available 43 years ago, so the obvious investigation was a plain X-ray (previous barium enemas had been reported as normal). The X-ray indicated the presence of an abnormal shadow suggestive of a foreign body. This made sense so we organised a laparotomy and not surprisingly found the corrugated drain tubing left accidentally following the cholecystectomy. (Refer to Figure 6.1, centre insert page 3.) The thought of litigation did not cross his mind such was the prevailing attitude at the time and the particular nature of the relieved person.

DISCUSSION AND LESSONS LEARNED

- It is usually possible to evaluate the genuineness of your patient by their personality and demeanour. However, all patients should be considered as having a genuine problem until proved otherwise, and managed accordingly.
- Recurrent incomplete small bowel obstruction showing transient episodes of obstructive symptoms often do not have all classic symptoms or signs present. Abdominal signs may be unremarkable and self-limiting.
- Adhesional abdominal pain is very difficult to diagnose and is a diagnosis of exclusion.
- The plain X-ray is still a valuable and effective investigation and often underused.

A lost cause is a lost testicle

The mother of Greg N, aged 15, rang to say that he was complaining of severe suprapubic pain following its sudden onset. After an hour the pain was also in his right groin and he had vomited three times. I instructed her to bring Greg to the office, adding that acute appendicitis or a strangulated hernia should be excluded. On examination the right testicle was tender, red and swollen. Its elevation increased the pain. I rang the nearest surgeon and asked him to attend to this torsion of the testis, adding that its onset would be three hours by the time he saw the patient. He readily agreed.

Diagnosis and outcome

The surgeon rang me some seven hours later saying that he had to perform orchidectomy because the testicle was infarcted. I was not surprised but was very disappointed at his error of judgement.

DISCUSSION AND LESSONS LEARNED

- Early operation with testicular torsion is imperative, because if the testis is deprived of its blood supply for more than a few hours infarction is inevitable and excision becomes necessary. My working rule is surgical intervention within four hours. Rates of testicular salvage are dependent on the time from the start of symptoms until surgery—within four to six hours, 100 per cent of torsive testes are salvageable, but by 12 hours the salvage rate has dropped to 20 per cent.

- Torsion of the testis can present as lower abdominal or suprapubic pain rather than simply testicular or scrotal pain.
- Excluding mumps, no youth under the age of 18 years with severe testicular pain should be diagnosed as acute epididymo-orchitis until the testis has been exposed at operation and torsion excluded. Many testes are lost because of inappropriate delays with referral for an ultrasound. The patient should be referred immediately to a surgeon or surgical centre (Bird, 2003).
- In country practice I learned to perform the simple operation rather than having to send such cases to a distant surgeon for management. No more infarcted testes!

Ignorance is not bliss

Julie V, aged 6, was enjoying her summer vacation at a seaside resort when she developed severe central abdominal pain and vomiting.

The following sad story is presented in chronological sequence.

Day 1: Sudden onset of central to lower abdominal pain and vomiting. Patient looked pale.

Day 2: Abdominal pain and vomiting persisted; difficulty in walking, febrile. Patient appeared very sick and pale. The doctor made a home visit, took her temperature and palpated her abdomen. 'It could be appendicitis but it's probably gastroenteritis. I'll prescribe antibiotics and she should settle.'

Day 3 am: Abdominal pain now very severe; vomiting and fever worse. Diarrhoea developed and Julie was too sick to get up. The doctor explained over the phone, 'The diarrhoea is due to the antibiotics. I'll prescribe an antidiarrhoea mixture'.

Day 3 pm: Mother phoned the doctor to say how concerned she was because Julie was getting worse by the hour. She asked whether Julie should be taken to hospital. 'It's not necessary. They'd only do what you're already doing at home.'

Day 4 (Saturday) am: Patient worse: very pale; diarrhoea now almost continuous. Mother visited doctor's surgery and was told, 'These gastro things can go on for a few days'.

Day 4 pm: Parents took Julie to a base hospital about 30 km away. The casualty doctor diagnosed acute appendicitis and peritonitis. At surgery a perforated gangrenous appendix was removed and a pelvic abscess drained.

Day 10: Julie was discharged home, very lethargic and weak with residual abdominal pain.

Day 12: Julie developed abdominal pain, fever, nausea and diarrhoea. I was called to see her for the first time. Examination revealed a tender abdomen and a tender boggy mass was palpable *per rectum.* A diagnosis of pelvic abscess was made and the patient was hospitalised under the care of her surgeon.

Days 13–18: Pain, fever, nausea and diarrhoea persisted. Conservative treatment was given but the patient grew weak and wasted.

Day 19: Spontaneous discharge of pus *per rectum* relieved her symptoms over the next two days.

Days 22–41: Julie went home and gradually improved, despite intermittent bouts of colicky abdominal pain.

Days 42–151: Julie was very healthy and normal, free of abdominal pain.

Day 152 (Sunday): Julie had a sudden bout of agonising abdominal pain followed by vomiting. As I was unavailable at the time, the locum service was contacted. A young locum appeared at the door of the house and was told the history, with the suggestion that this new development could be related to the previous illness. 'Do you want me to stay or go?' he asked. He stayed and examined Julie's ears and throat; palpated her abdomen; and asked her to walk, hop on one leg and then jump. (She failed the latter tests.) He then announced confidently, 'There's absolutely nothing wrong—she's possibly coming down with a gastro thing. That will be $90.00'. All in three minutes!

Day 153: The patient remained in bed, sleeping almost constantly and moaning occasionally with pain. She had no bowel movement. Her temperature started to rise in the evening and she grew pale.

Day 154: She developed very severe pain and had a possible haematemesis at 1 am. She was visited by her regular doctor and admitted to hospital at once. After several hours of resuscitation in intensive care, being treated with intravenous fluids and antibiotics, she was taken to theatre for a laparotomy. A loop of small bowel, obstructed by adhesions, was found to be gangrenous and perforated leading to blood-stained faecal peritonitis. The section of bowel was removed, an end-to-end anastomosis performed, and the abdominal cavity carefully cleansed with cephazolin solution.

Days 155–180: Julie had a long convalescence in hospital with treatment for a subphrenic and a pelvic abscess.

For the next 12 years, Julie continued to have problems after further surgery for adhesions and intra-abdominal abscesses. Medical litigation was instituted and a settlement was eventually reached. Now, as an adult, her main problem is sub-fertility.

DISCUSSION AND LESSONS LEARNED

- Appendicitis should never be underestimated, especially in young children. It should be foremost in mind when 'gastroenteritis' appears to be getting worse.
- A rushed physical examination, especially in the home, can be full of hazards. In particular the all-important rectal examination gets neglected.
- In this case the previous history appears to have been ignored. Any current illness should always be assessed within the context of the past history.
- The importance of continuing care by the same doctor is obvious. Perhaps we should make ourselves more accessible after hours to these patients and families.
- We should be considerate of the difficult position of parents with sick children and be sensitive to pleas for help. Unfortunately, the many anxious calls for help in this case resulted in angry responses.
- It's easy to be wise after the event.

The need for X-ray vision

Case 1

Danny, aged 8, presented with three days of pain in his foot causing a limp. His mother said he was complaining of the pain when he was preparing for school, which he dislikes, especially on athletics days. She thought that this was the reason for his complaint and ignored it initially. Danny insisted that the pain came on suddenly when he was running around the house. On examination there was no swelling but deep tenderness over the middle of the sole of the foot adjacent to the base of the second metatarsal.

An X-ray revealed a snapped-off needle embedded in Danny's foot (Figure 6.2). Danny proudly displayed the piece of metal removed from a bloodless foot under general anaesthesia, while his poor mother, upset at her misjudgement, required soothing empathy from a parent of five children.

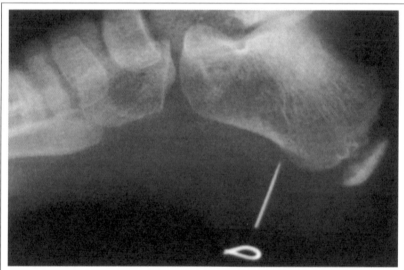

Fig. 6.2 X-ray of Danny's foot showing the embedded needle

Case 2

Angela, a 66-year-old Italian lady, presented with a four-day history of a very painful knee. It was red and tender over the prepatella bursa, causing her so much discomfort that her relatives brought her in a wheelchair. I referred her immediately to an orthopaedic surgeon in the adjoining medical centre. He contacted me with the news that she had prepatella bursitis due to bacterial infection; he had prescribed flucloxacillin and sent her home. Two days later she presented to Alan, one of my colleagues, claiming that the problem was worse.

An X-ray of the knee revealed a broken needle in the soft tissues over the knee. Red faces all around, but Alan sported a grin like a Cheshire cat for a long time. Angela, incidentally, was an avid seamstress. She gave us no history of a sharp pain while kneeling on the floor.

Case 3

Ron, aged 48, was a farmer who loved tinkering in his large workshop. One day while oxywelding, gunpowder exploded causing burns to exposed parts of his body, especially to his face. (Refer to Figure 6.3, centre insert page 3.) His appearance was quite dramatic but the burns settled and eventually healed nicely. I initially checked his eyes, which he claimed were uncomfortable, and found a considerable amount of grit, charcoal and inflammation. After I removed the debris, he said that the eyes felt better but that the right eye was sore and slightly blurred. I reassured him that it was the effects of the burns. However, when this persisted, I asked for an ophthalmologist's opinion. The eye was X-rayed and an intraocular metallic foreign body was found.

Case 4

Bruce, aged 21, a prisoner on parole, presented one evening with lacerations to the wrist caused by a jagged bottle used in a fight at a hotel. I explored and cleaned the wounds, which seemed generally clean, and sutured them. On review for suture removal, he complained that the main wound was very sore but I reassured him and explained that it was a deep wound. Some weeks later the medical officer attached to the prison rang me to say that he had removed a 1–2 cm fragment of glass from the wound, after identifying it on X-ray when the patient complained of persistent pain. He added that the patient was not impressed. I still feel uneasy!

DISCUSSION AND LESSONS LEARNED

- If in any doubt, X-ray, especially in the context of a litigation-conscious public. Mandatory X-rays for foreign bodies include the feet of limping children, injured areas where exploding glass or metal is involved, especially the eyes, gunshot wounds and similar trauma.
- Most glass is radio-opaque and so wounds caused by glass—including motor accidents—demand an X-ray even after careful exploration. Ultra-sound imaging is a reliable option. Failure to identify a foreign body in a wound can have severe consequences, especially in diabetic patients.

X-rays and human error

Thomas H, a 54-year-old warehouse manager in good general health, presented with an eight-week history of low-back pain without sciatica.

He described the pain as a deep ache that is present day and night and getting worse. It was aggravated by activity including walking and jogging, and the only relief was provided by analgesics taken orally. He observed that he had become progressively lethargic over the past few months and had lost about 2 kg. He admitted to the presence of a smoker's cough caused by smoking '20 cigarettes daily since he was a lad' but denied chest pain, dyspnoea, wheezing or a productive cough.

Examination revealed a large, apparently fit man with the main abnormality being tenderness to digital palpation over the spinous process of L4. He had painful limitation of flexion, extension and lateral flexion (bilaterally) of his lumbar spine. There was a flattened lumbar lordosis, but the neurological examination of his lower limbs was normal. Examination of his chest, abdomen and rectum were normal.

Diagnosis

X-rays of his chest and lumbosacral spine were taken (Figure 6.4). The chest X-ray was reported as normal and his lumbosacral spinal X-ray report read:

> There is minor osteophytic lipping anteriorly and laterally
> in several of the discs but no disc space narrowing. The

*lower apophyseal joints exhibit a little degenerative
disease. No metastases are seen and there are no signs of
spondylolisthesis.*

When Thomas rang the clinic to discuss the results of the investigations
he was informed that the X-rays were normal and that there was nothing
to worry about. However, his back continued to ache and so he decided to
consult a non-medical health professional who, after seeing his X-rays, rang
our clinic to advise that the patient had a destructive lesion in the body of L4.

The X-rays were reviewed by the radiologist who then reported:

*A lytic lesion is present in the anterior aspect of the L4
vertebral body . . . the bone texture is otherwise normal.
Metastasis is the most likely cause for this lesion and less likely
is myeloma or a retroperitoneal lesion growing posteriorly.*

A carcinoma of the lung is the most likely primary that could cause this
metastatic lesion. Other primaries could arise from the kidney, adrenal, thyroid
and melanoma. The prostate causes osteosclerotic metastases to the spine.

A follow-up X-ray of the lung revealed a 2 cm mass in the right middle
lobe. At fibre-optic bronchoscopy there was an erythematous cobblestone
mucosal lesion in the right middle lobe bronchus. Brushing, washings
and biopsies were taken but the results were inconclusive. However, the
carcinoma eventually became obvious with time.

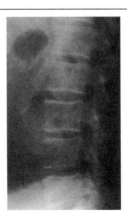

Fig. 6.4 X-ray of lumbar spine of Thomas H

DISCUSSION AND LESSONS LEARNED

- It is important to back one's clinical judgement. Any middle-aged or elderly patient presenting with back pain that is there day and night has a malignant disease until proved otherwise. A high index of suspicion demands complete and careful follow-through of the physical examination and appropriate investigations.
- X-rays of the chest and spine can appear quite normal in the early stages of malignant disease. If clinically appropriate, follow-up X-rays should be arranged, including bone scans.
- Similarly, investigations of the bronchial tree for malignant disease can be negative in the presence of malignant disease.
- Mistakes can be made by radiologists and by staff transcribing the report. Legally the responsibility for the patient may be shared by the radiologist and the referring doctor. If the X-rays are returned to general practitioners, it is valuable to review the films to the best of their ability before conveying the report to patients.

Are you playing Russian roulette with your patients?

The patient, a young woman, presented with the problem of wax in her right ear. It seemed a simple procedure but it suddenly went wrong. A highly unlikely malfunction with the standard syringe led to the violent projection of the syringe nozzle into the patient's auditory canal (Figures 6.5 and 6.6).

The threads at the base of the brass syringe were fine and worn presumably from previous assembly on the wrong threads. Combined with a less than smooth-flowing plunger, the sudden detachment resulted in the forward projection of the nozzle into the canal despite the use of a steadying extended small finger for stabilisation.

The patient was acutely distressed by the injury but once composed allowed inspection. There appeared to be a laceration of the canal with an intact drum.

On review the next day, however, the patient complained of deafness in the ear since the injury, a complaint that persisted despite further tentative enquiry at 70 decibels.

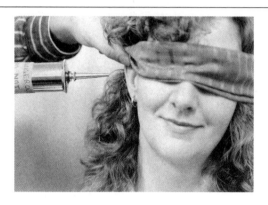

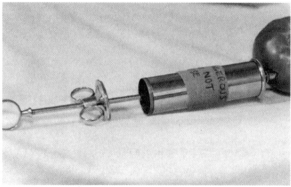

Fig. 6.5 and 6.6 Malfunction of a standard syringe led to the violent projection of the syringe nozzle into the patient's auditory canal

I feared my initial assessment may have been wishful thinking. Fortunately, however, an ENT opinion revealed a canal injury with an intact drum and the patient's hearing returned after clearing of the canal.

The use of a rounded nozzle may have prevented the gouging injury but at the expense of the nozzle sliding onwards and damaging the drum.

DISCUSSION AND LESSONS LEARNED

- Discussing this accident with colleagues, I found many were aware of the potential for injury with such syringes. I believe, in the interest of safety, the force that generates the hydrostatic pressure should be distant from the ear and the source of the stream should not be a rigid metal canula. I now use a plastic 20 mL syringe with the plastic tubing from a standard 'butterfly' or winged infusion set. Systems such as a foot pump give the operator the advantage of a free hand when syringing.

- Medical negligence claims and complaints against GPs and their staff because of ear syringing do occur. The reasons and percentages of claims are: poor technique (43%), faulty equipment (26%), excessive pressure (26%), failure to examine the ear before syringing (5%) (Bird, 2008).

Underestimating motor mower power

Case 1

A 42-year-old patient of mine presented to the emergency department of a base hospital with lacerations to the first and second toes of his right foot, sustained from a rotary motor mower while he was mowing the long grass in his mother's backyard. The wounds were debrided, sutured and dressed. He was given an injection of tetanus toxoid and oral tetracyclines.

Four days later he presented to me complaining of severe pain in his foot. The wounds were inflamed and swollen. I took an X-ray, which revealed fractures of three phalanges of these toes and foreign bodies in the wound. He was taken to theatre where, under general anaesthetic, the wound was reopened, and dirt and small stones removed. The wound was left open for some days before eventual closure. Penicillin was the antibiotic of choice.

Outcome

The wound appeared to heal nicely but the patient presented later with suppuration and pain. X-rays confirmed osteomyelitis in the proximal phalanx of his great toe.

Case 2

Mark T, a 23-year-old council gardener, presented with a painful swollen right thigh following an injury 11 days before. While using a rotary motor mower, he was struck sharply on the inner mid-thigh by an object considered to be a stone. The pain was intense and weight bearing on that leg was impossible. He visited a nearby medical centre and was advised to apply ice packs, and then rest and elevate the leg. The pain became worse and he attended again but was given ultrasound therapy and crutches.

When I eventually saw him, he was in severe pain from a swollen red right thigh in which a 5 mm long wound was noted. An X-ray revealed a piece of wire within the thigh with extensive gas formation, confirming the presence of a foreign body with gas gangrene (Figure 6.7). He was sent immediately to a specialist unit for extensive surgery; he was fortunate to survive as he developed shock and required several days in intensive care.

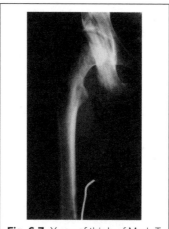

Fig. 6.7 X-ray of thigh of Mark T

DISCUSSION AND LESSONS LEARNED

- A tremendous amount of energy is transmitted to the limb from the blades of the mower and the full extent of the injury, especially fractures to adjacent bone, is not apparent. It is likely that foreign bodies have been

introduced, and such direct injuries should be treated as a compound
fracture from the outset. An X-ray is mandatory.
- Since these machines are capable of propelling objects at high velocity, all
possible penetrating injuries should be X-rayed.
- These cases of osteomyelitis, gas gangrene and wound infection highlight
the problem of early mismanagement.

Beware children and needle-sticks

After a man whom I suspected was an IV drug user left my office, I noticed
a used needle and syringe on his seat. Intending to use this as evidence of his
IV drug use (which he denied), I decided to keep the needle and syringe.

I left it in an adjacent room. To my horror a small child came into my
office, climbed up and pricked himself with the needle.

I had to explain to his mother that the needle was from a suspected IV
drug user and that the child needed to have blood tests to determine if he had
contracted an infectious disease such as hepatitis B, hepatitis C and HIV. The
outcome was satisfactory but it was very distressing to all concerned.

DISCUSSION AND LESSONS LEARNED
- It is vital to dispose of needle-sticks and other sharps quickly and
effectively in a secure container.
- Special care is needed where children are active and it is important for
parents and staff to keep them under constant surveillance in the surgery.
- For a needle-stick injury, immediate diplomatic counselling of the exposed
person and family (with careful follow-up) is mandatory.

Red faces

The prescription pad

My young medical colleague in a city practice had just completed writing a pad prescription for an oral contraceptive for a woman who infrequently came to the practice. My colleague noted that she had not had a Pap smear for three years and she willingly agreed that in the presence of the practice nurse she would have one now. My young colleague went to fetch the nurse and noted that a man was having an unusual type of convulsion on the floor of the waiting room. He administered necessary first aid to the young man, who then stood up and seemed perfectly lucid and well. My colleague's Pap smear patient suddenly rushed from the examination room where she had been left on the couch during this man's alleged convulsion, grabbed him by the arm, dashed out of the door and was never to be seen again.

Two hours later, two separate pharmacists phoned my young colleague to enquire whether the amounts of opioids written on his prescriptions for this young woman and the alleged epileptic were indeed correct. My young colleague then noted that five pages had been removed from the back of his prescription pad. The oral contraceptive script of course already had his signature on it, and this had been forged onto the stolen prescription pages.

DISCUSSION AND LESSONS LEARNED

- This situation would be unlikely to occur if prescriptions were generated electronically; indeed, the young colleague's practice has used the electronic system ever since.

- Prescription pads are frequently stolen in toto from clinics, and drug abusers have learnt every conceivable method of obtaining these, including my colleague's non-epileptic young man.
- Many practices including this one keep a list of drugs of habitation and addiction, which doctors in the practice refuse to supply to patients except those known to be genuine medical users rather than possible abusers.
- Other items of medical equipment are frequently stolen (in addition to the clinic's magazines!) and syringes and needles particularly should be kept securely.

Tonsillitis: traps for the unwary

In country practice I had acquired the skills for tonsillectomy, a much over-performed operation in past years. A colleague from another country practice referred to me a 20-year-old woman for tonsillectomy. I thought that the tonsils were normal, but both he and the patient insisted they should be removed because of a recent shocking attack of tonsillitis. I obliged.

A few months later he rang saying he had a 23-year-old woman with another terrible bout of tonsillitis. This seemed most unusual and so I requested to see the patient the following day. Indeed she did have severe tonsillitis, but she also had petechiae on the soft palate, widespread lymphadenopathy, splenomegaly and a positive Paul–Bunnell test. (Refer to Figure 7.1, centre insert page 4.)

I knew these things because I had been 'caught out' giving penicillin and ampicillin to patients for acute tonsillitis (streptococcal I thought!) only to have severe maculopapular rashes develop.

DISCUSSION AND LESSONS LEARNED

- At least 50 per cent of patients with Epstein–Barr mononucleosis develop tonsillitis with a profuse whitish-yellow exudate. It can be easily confused with bacterial tonsillitis.

- We had not been taught this information and pitfall in medical school. It just shows the importance of basic knowledge, and what you do not know you simply mismanage. Our undergraduate training seemed to program us for high-technology hospital-based medicine—prepared us for the zoo and not the jungle so to speak. We have to work towards correcting this nonsense.

Vaginal tamponade

One evening an 18-year-old woman presented to the emergency room of our hospital complaining of an offensive vaginal discharge. Offensive was an understatement! Further questioning established that it was possibly a retained vaginal tampon and sex had impacted it further.

I could readily see the tampon and removed it with sponge-holding forceps. The odour was overbearing and I staggered with weak knees to the toilet to dispose of the putrid object. An embarrassing stench (especially for the patient) pervaded that area of the hospital. I then mentally devised a scheme to make the procedure more aesthetic for all concerned.

The patient contacted me two days later to say that the problem persisted. I examined her again and there was another tampon and the same mousy discharge. I felt most embarrassed about being 'overcome' by the previous consultation and not checking that the vagina was 'all clear'. This time I brought a plastic bucket of water to the introitus and plunged the tampon (still attached to the forceps) into the bucket. After checking that the vagina was empty I sped to the toilet, tipped the water and the tampon into the slush bowl and flushed it. Virtually no smell this time.

DISCUSSION AND LESSONS LEARNED

- I always make sure that no other foreign bodies remain after one is removed from the body, especially from the vagina and rectum, which seem to be repositories for all types of weird and wonderful objects these days. Removing vibrators from both is not uncommon, but the most unusual and difficult object extracted was an alarm clock from the rectum of an army fellow.

- It is important not to further humiliate patients who are already embarrassed by their predicament. The method of plunging the tampon under water works beautifully and does not create smells in the treatment area. This bucket-of-water method also works for removing impacted faeces.

Big-headed and pig-headed

One of the liabilities for general practitioners in the day-to-day practice of their art is a direct consequence of one of the greatest assets of general practice—continuing care. When we see the same patient year in and year out—perhaps even 10 or 12 times a year—subtle changes in the patient are not noticed and are often camouflaged by a host of previously diagnosed neurotic symptoms. We are all aware that one day we will miss something important that the outsider—the consultant, the locum, the intern or even the student—will detect instantly. We hope that this will not occur too often and pray that the outcome of our delayed diagnosis will not be sinister. This case illustrates such an occurrence.

Miss Davies, a 68-year-old woman, had attended our clinic for 25 years and had been seeing me for almost six of those years. She had a history of cholelithiasis and reflux oesophagitis, and about two years ago had complained of neck pain and headaches. I had X-rayed her neck and found the usual spondyloarthritic changes to be expected in a patient of this age. The neural foramina were encroached on by osteophytes at C2 to 3, C3 to 4 and C6 to 7.

For the next two years I confidently and graciously explained away her neck pain and headache in terms of these changes. Then a final-year medical student was attached to our practice for two weeks and I asked her to interview Miss Davies, warning the student that she probably would hear a barrage of complaints about neck pain and headache. I allowed the student

10 minutes and then walked into the room and said somewhat sardonically, 'Well, what did you discover?'

'Don't you think her head looks a little large?' she replied. 'Do you think she might have Paget's disease?'

'Oh no,' I retorted, 'Miss Davies has always looked like this.'

At this stage the patient interjected, 'You know, Doctor, I've always been worried about getting Paget's disease: my father died of it.'

'Well, Miss Davies,' I replied, 'Paget's disease, to the best of my knowledge, is not hereditary but to reassure you I'll order a skull X-ray.' The result of the X-ray: florid Paget's disease.

DISCUSSION AND LESSONS LEARNED
- Try to treat each new complaint as if it were occurring in a new patient.
- Try to divorce yourself from your knowledge of the patient's premorbid personality in assessing this new complaint.
- Investigate the complaint and treat it appropriately, and then bring it into the context of overall management of the patient.
- If the patient reports changes in her or his appearance, ask for old photographs with which to compare her or his present appearance—especially in suspected endocrine conditions such as myxoedema, Cushing's syndrome and acromegaly.

Six years of unnecessary nocturnal hell

Bernard is a keen sportsman who unfortunately suffered with severe pain around his right ankle for six long years until the elusive diagnosis was made and an instant cure provided. He was 34 years old when he first presented with the pain, which developed insidiously.

He consulted a rheumatologist who said that he had post-traumatic arthritis and that an X-ray that reported 'some spurring on the dorsal surface of the neck and body of the right talus' was of little significance (Figure 7.2).

Bernard first consulted me about 12 months after his problem started, when the pain became very severe, causing him sleepless nights unless he took non-steroidal anti-inflammatory drugs (NSAIDs). He described the pain as feeling 'as though there was a nerve on edge' but said the aspirin was very effective for pain relief. On examination of his right ankle there was acute localised tenderness on the anteromedial aspect of his ankle with some diffuse area of soft tissue swelling. The ankle joint was stable, and all movements and gait were normal. I referred him to an orthopaedic surgeon who was an expert on ankle disorders.

Surgery

The surgeon found a large area of discoloured irregular-looking synovitis with bone erosions on both the talus and the anterior tibia. He said the diagnosis was uncertain and performed localised synovectomy, which was reported as 'non-specific chronic synovitis'.

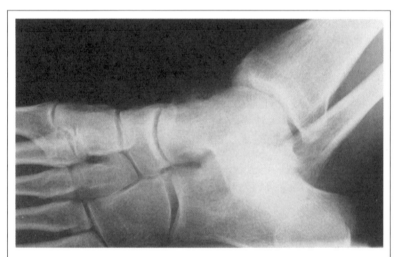

Fig. 7.2 Plain X-ray of Bernard's foot. Note the osteophytic reaction on the anteromedial aspect of the talus with radiolucent areas

Post-surgical progress

Bernard's pain continued relentlessly. The surgeon felt Bernard should be fine, but further visits to his rheumatologist did not help. The latter performed several tests including full blood examination (FBE), ESR, rheumatoid arthritis factor, uric acid, tissue typing and plain X-rays, all of which were reported as normal. Bernard was told that he had 'a low-grade inflammatory joint disease, most likely of rheumatoid variation' and that he would have to learn to live with it with the help of the effective NSAIDs. However, he battled on bravely even with the label of 'neurotic', which he himself was beginning to believe. Acupuncture and various other remedies were ineffective.

Five years later

When I met Bernard socially five years later, I was distressed to discover that in addition to his painful ankle he had a severe duodenal ulcer that was responsible for melaenas. He said that the ankle pain was worse than ever, especially at night. It was intense first thing in the morning when he put his foot to the floor. He then hobbled around for 15 minutes, but it did not bother him much during the day when he was occupied and busy.

'Light switch' and the solution

Something suddenly clicked in the sluggish grey matter. Could it be? I rang another orthopaedic surgeon and, yes, he thought an osteoid osteoma was a definite possibility. We organised a bone scan that showed a hot spot in the neck of the talus 'suggestive of an osteoid osteoma'.

At surgery, bone chiselling revealed the seemingly innocent little tumour that caused so much pain—the osteoma with its cherry red soft core about 8 mm in diameter. It was removed and the defect packed with bone wax.

Bernard has lived and slept happily ever after. Well almost! The epigastric pain of his old NSAID-induced peptic ulcer still reminds him of six years of relative hell!

DISCUSSION AND LESSONS LEARNED

- Osteoid osteomas are nasty little tumours that test the diagnostic acumen of the practitioner mainly because they are rare. As a rule they affect older children and adolescents, and males are affected twice as often as females. The pain is not relieved by rest but classically by aspirin. Any bone (except those of the skull) can be affected but the tibia and the femur are the main targets.

- Patients complaining of chronic pain can be readily labelled as functional. Somehow these patients believe they harbour a tumour and failure to diagnose the tumour makes us look professionally incompetent. As Bailey (1960) puts it: 'In mild or early cases the pain occasioned by this condition is often attributed to a neurosis'.

- Careful note should be taken of any abnormal X-ray signs, especially with a persistent clinical problem. The radiological changes (sclerotic lesion with radiolucent centre) were present but ignored.

- Some degree of surgical intervention tends to make us complacent that we have a definitive answer to the problem.

- Long-term NSAIDs are a hazard, as is well illustrated with this patient.

- The next time around we hope we will all pick the osteoid osteoma. Or will we? As our surgeon said: 'Always think of an osteoid osteoma in a young lad with unusual pain in a leg (especially pain that responds nicely to aspirin or paracetamol)'.

Watching your P's and cues

Sheryl was a cheerful and apparently healthy 31-year-old nurse who had recently assumed nursing duties at our hospital, having worked in various centres while travelling around Australia over the past 12 years.

She soon presented with severe lower abdominal pain. I noted that her behaviour was somewhat bizarre. She was whimpering, agitated and writhing with severe colicky pain and vomiting. Examination revealed multiple scars on her distended abdomen, mild generalised tenderness and increased bowel sounds. The rectum was empty. She produced a letter outlining that she had suffered multiple bouts of severe abdominal pain, which had resulted in a total of 17 surgical procedures including an appendicectomy, a cholecystectomy, Billroth II gastrectomy, two ovarian cystectomies, hysterectomy, splenectomy, division of adhesions for bowel obstruction and several exploratory laparotomies. She was 'allergic' to pentazocine, morphine, barbiturates and codeine; pethidine was 'the only effective treatment for the attack'.

Diagnosis

My immediate diagnosis was pethidine addiction, although Munchausen syndrome or bowel obstruction secondary to adhesions were possibilities. Management in hospital included an intravenous drip, nasogastric suction and chlorpromazine 25 mg by intramuscular injection. (Refer to Figure 7.3, centre insert page 4.) A plain X-ray of her abdomen showed no abnormalities. Several hours later when she felt comfortable a nurse reported that a urine specimen left on the bench was coloured red but negative for blood. The penny dropped!

DISCUSSION AND LESSONS LEARNED

- Intermittent porphyria should be considered in such patients. Sheryl had a typical history of this rare disorder. Onset is approximately at age 20 and the patient is asymptomatic for long periods. It mimics bowel obstruction, although psychiatric disturbances are manifested during 'attacks', and it is responsive to chlorpromazine. Urine usually is colourless but turns red on exposure to sunlight.
- These patients are often subjected to multiple abdominal surgical procedures and often diagnosed as pethidine addicts as I had initially thought with Sheryl.

He needed surgery like a hole in the head

The afternoon consultation was interrupted by a phone call from a local farmer describing a motor vehicle accident near his farmhouse. The driver had been injured when his car left the road and crashed into a tree.

At the scene of the accident a blood-spattered middle-aged man was stumbling around, apparently intoxicated but not smelling of alcohol. There were several lacerations on his scalp and face but otherwise he seemed free from injury. His somewhat irrational behaviour made it difficult to obtain a history.

The ambulance arrived and we decided to send him to the nearest base hospital, about 80 km away. I phoned the admitting officer in advance to tell him that George (aged about 40), who was unknown to us, had sustained head injuries. By the time the ambulance reached the hospital the patient was comatose and unresponsive to verbal commands.

Provisional diagnosis

George was assessed by a surgeon who diagnosed an extradural haematoma and organised its urgent decompression.

Tension mounted as the unconscious patient was rushed to theatre, his wounds cleaned and his head shaved (a gleaming dome awaiting the surgical assault). The anaesthetist inserted an intravenous line while, in the wings of the operating theatre, the impatient and anxious surgeon waited to snatch yet another patient from the jaws of death. Then, as the surgical drama was about to unfold, the drapes began to stir and the patient roused from his afternoon 'slumber'. Sitting upright on the operating table, he gazed around in bewilderment, and then began to deliver an emotional verbal assault punctuated by the 'great Australian adjective'.

The bemused surgeon, known for his ability to have the 'last word', turned to the theatre sister with, 'Is there an item number for a head shave?'

Revised diagnosis

The patient was a type 1 diabetic; that afternoon he had been hypoglycaemic. It took only 100 mL of the 5 per cent intravenous dextrose routinely administered by the anaesthetist to correct the dangerously low blood sugar level.

DISCUSSION AND LESSONS LEARNED

- Any patient found unconscious should be regarded as hypoglycaemic (especially when he or she is unknown to the doctor) until proved otherwise. A blood glucose estimation takes about two minutes.
- In dealing with accidents, especially those in unusual circumstances, we should ask ourselves, 'What really caused this accident: alcohol, drugs or a medical emergency (such as epilepsy, hypoglycaemia, cerebrovascular accident, myocardial infarction)?'

- The case highlights the importance of searching the patient for evidence of a medical condition such as diabetes or epilepsy and the value of wearing medical identity discs.

Confidentiality owed to a dog

For several years, 80-year-old Mary had seen her GP every week. She walked to the practice with her dog, and tied the dog to the gate at the front of the practice during her visit.

One morning there was a loud commotion outside the practice. A mother rushed into the waiting room with her three-year-old child who had been bitten on the leg by Mary's dog (one of the other patients later reported that she saw the child kick the dog, thus provoking the attack). The GP immediately took the child to the treatment room to deal with the dog bite. In the interim, Mary slipped out of the practice, quickly untied her dog and went home.

The mother of the child was furious and wanted to report the dog to the local council to have it destroyed. She demanded that the GP give her the name and address of the patient so that she could make the notification to the council.

The GP was not sure what she should do and contacted her medical defence organisation. The GP was advised that a duty of confidentiality was owed to the patient (and her dog) and she should politely inform the mother that she was unable to give her this information.

The GP did not hear anything further about the matter. Mary continued to attend the practice each week, but she left her dog at home.

DISCUSSION AND LESSONS LEARNED
- Doctors have both a legal and professional duty to protect patient confidentiality and privacy.
- Doctors can provide information to a third party in limited circumstances, such as when:

- the patient consents to the release of the information
- disclosure is made to another health practitioner to ensure the appropriate medical care of the patient
- disclosure is required by or under law or a court/tribunal order, e.g. mandatory reporting of child abuse, a subpoena or search warrant
- there is an overriding duty in the public interest to disclose information, such as to prevent a serious threat to the life, health or safety of a patient or another person, and it is unreasonable or impracticable to obtain the patient's consent, e.g. a patient who refuses to stop driving despite medical advice to do so, or a patient who threatens harm against another person.

- In this case, none of the exceptions to the duty of confidentiality and privacy applied—the patient did not want her contact details disclosed to the child's mother and there was no public interest in doing so.

Wrong number!

Andrew, four years of age, was brought to the practice by his mother with pain and swelling of his penis. The GP examined the child and was concerned that he may have paraphimosis. The GP rang the children's hospital to obtain advice about whether the patient needed to be urgently transferred to hospital. The surgical registrar asked the GP to take a photo of the penis and send it to her to assess whether it was a genuine paraphimosis, or the less serious phimosis.

The GP obtained the mother's permission and assistance to take a photo of the child's penis using his mobile phone. The GP then sent the photo, with a message 'pending U/A' (urinalysis).

The GP received a call a few minutes later from a man asking why a photo of a penis had been sent to him. The GP immediately realised he must have sent the photo to the wrong number. He apologised profusely and explained he was a doctor who was trying to diagnose a medical condition. The GP asked the man to immediately delete the photo, which he agreed to do.

The GP explained the situation to the mother and apologised for the error. He re-checked the surgical registrar's phone number, finding he had transcribed one digit incorrectly. He sent the photo to the registrar and subsequently obtained advice that it was not a surgical emergency.

One month later, the police attended the GP's home. The police informed the GP that a complaint had been made by a member of the public that he had electronically transmitted child pornography. The GP confirmed he was a doctor and explained the error to the police. Fortunately, the police were satisfied with his explanation. They said they would report back to the Police Child Abuse Squad and the investigation would be closed.

DISCUSSION AND LESSONS LEARNED

- The use of clinical photography is becoming more widespread in clinical practice.
- Key medico-legal issues to consider are:
    - whether an image is appropriate and adequate for the provision of clinical care
    - whether consent has been given for the collection, use and disclosure of the image
    - how the clinical image should be retained and stored.
- In this case, the error could have been avoided if the GP had entered the phone number and sent a message to the surgical registrar asking her to confirm her identity before sending the photo, or asking the surgical registrar to ring the GP back and then send the photo to that number.

Picking up the pieces: the aftermaths of three deaths

'What is a myocardial infarction, Doctor?'

The receptionist told me a patient on the phone wished to speak to an independent doctor in our practice about an urgent problem. The distressed woman's opening words were: 'What is a myocardial infarction, Doctor? I simply have to speak to you about it; I'm too embarrassed to speak to the doctors there that I know'.

The story unfolded. Her husband, aged 56, had been treated by Dr A for hypertension. Her doctor was Dr B. Twelve months ago Dr C saw her husband at home early one morning because he had chest pain. Despite attempted resuscitation after a cardiac arrest in the ambulance, he was dead on arrival at the hospital.

Everything happened so suddenly that she did not have an opportunity to speak to a doctor at the time but assumed her husband died from a heart attack. However, a copy of the death certificate that stated death was caused by 'myocardial infarction' confused her. She had mulled over this for the past year. Her catharsis began: 'How could he have died in this modern day of wonder medicine? Why didn't Dr A warn us this could happen? If only I could have spoken to one of the doctors. If only I'd known exactly how he died. I have felt like killing myself, I've been so depressed. I feel so bad about the way I looked after him'.

An erroneous death certificate

A patient consulted me last year, distressed and angry about the death certificate issued after her husband's death. She said, 'This certificate is wrong. It's an illegal document. It's a lie—Ted did not die from septicaemia after bronchopneumonia—he had a heart attack.'

Ted, who had a history of ischaemic heart disease, was found semiconscious with a blood pressure of 80/40 and a temperature of 38 °C. When hospitalised, with a provisional diagnosis of septicaemia, he was treated with intravenous antibiotics. He developed heart failure and died 48 hours later; the resident doctor issued the death certificate. Later, a postmortem revealed an extensive myocardial infarction.

Her grief and hostility towards the doctors at the hospital were profound. 'Doctor, the diagnosis is wrong. The treatment was wrong—you will have to change it.'

The unreal image of the great hospital

'Doctor, would you please call on Mum? She is in a terrible state over Dad's death, although it was four months ago.'

Dad was a 72-year-old farmer who developed pyloric stenosis after a long history of peptic ulceration. He was admitted to a major teaching hospital in the city, under the care of a surgeon. His postoperative course had been good until a tear developed in the lower oesophagus following an episode of vomiting. After a high spinal anaesthetic on his third visit to the theatre, he became hypotensive and was admitted to the intensive care unit, where he died 16 days later.

When I called to see his widow I was taken into the dining room. A mass of medical bills was spread out on the table and several relatives looked on solemnly. The sum of the accounts was astounding and made me aware of my ignorance of some aspects of the health system. Apart from the surgeon's bill, there were bills from the surgeon's assistant, the anaesthetist and the director of intensive care (51 items), and five other consultant visits that totalled a substantial sum. The hospital services included haematology, biochemistry, radiology (including 28 chest X-rays), and microbiology (80 items). With other services, including bed charges, the grand total was more than $105 000.

'Doctor, how could he have possibly died after all this expert care, in this day and age? What went wrong? Why do they send all these bills?' They were pensioners but, acting on my advice, had obtained private health insurance.

Counselling was almost impossible. Depression, grief and anger dominated the family's emotions. The breakthrough was a special visit to the family in the country by the surgeon. He explained what had happened and why modern technology and skilled medical practitioners could not save their husband and father.

DISCUSSIONS AND LESSONS LEARNED

- Better communication from all involved in patient care is essential for the resolution of grief and for the enhancement of the medical profession's image.
- It is important that grieving relatives know the exact cause of death. The role of the family doctor in explaining the details in a diplomatic, caring way cannot be overstated.
- Impromptu house calls, especially if the death was unexpected, would really help relatives to cope with their grief.
- The sending of large medical bills to grieving families is a complex issue. Some doctors make a policy of never doing so under such circumstances.
- As Hippocrates reminded us: 'Cure sometimes, treat often, comfort always'.
- Relatives place far more importance on the content of the death certificate than we appreciate. The Medical Certificate Cause of Death (the 'death certificate') is an important legal document. Accurate cause of death information is important for:
    - legal purposes, e.g. the information may be relevant to the determination of validity of a will, especially if dementia is listed on the certificate, or a life insurance payment
    - statistical and public health purposes—death certificates are the major source of Australia's mortality statistics

> – family members—to know what caused the death and to be aware of conditions that may occur in other family members.

- The death certification process is also an important safeguard against the disposal of bodies without professional scrutiny of the requirement for further investigation by the coroner, particularly in relation to suspicious deaths or where the cause of death is unknown. The need for public confidence in the death certification process was highlighted by the investigation into the actions of British GP Dr Harold Shipman, who was convicted of murdering 15 of his patients.
- Patients tend to hold the general practitioner responsible for the quality of the consultant care they receive; if dissatisfied, they often point an accusing finger at the referring doctor.
- We should be aware of the cost of specialist services and hospital charges, forewarn our patients about the likely ramifications and, if we have options, make referral decisions on the basis of their health insurance and financial resources.

The kernel of the tragedy

Neil was one of my first patients when I commenced general practice in the country. He was an athletic man of 22 years, more than 190 cm tall, and already married with a baby son.

The problem with which he presented was a 10-month history of persistent headaches early in the morning, increasing in severity and now waking him. The headache was dull in nature and, although diffuse, was mainly occipital in site. It was aggravated by coughing, sneezing and straining at the toilet. It was relieved by aspirin and tended to abate during the day. Associated with this were problems of dizziness when arising, and vomiting during the week that preceded this initial consultation. He had visited two doctors several times and they believed that the problem was related to stress and possibly to a previous neck injury. During the past six months he had been receiving chiropractic treatment.

Diagnosis

A provisional diagnosis of an intracerebral tumour was made and this was supported by the presence of papilloedema upon the ophthalmoscopic examination of his ocular fundus.

He was referred to a neurologist and investigations confirmed the presence of a space-occupying lesion in the left temporal lobe. During surgery a large inoperable astrocytoma was found. It was biopsied and as much as possible was excised. A course of radiotherapy began after the operation.

When Neil arrived home, the community was stunned to see the zombie-like man with his stark, shaven and scarred head bearing testimony to invasive and futile medical intervention. His young wife and his family were shattered by the death sentence coldly conveyed by the neurosurgeon: 'There is nothing further we can do; he has about three months left—possibly six at the most'.

The week of his return I was called urgently to his home to find him still in the throes of a grand mal convulsion. Intravenous diazepam was necessary to terminate the problem and subsequently phenytoin sodium was prescribed.

Immediately after his next outpatients review the family clan appeared on my doorstep—Mum, Dad, brothers and sisters. They were very angry and desperate. They said that they would try everything in their power and stated that they had made tentative arrangements to send Neil to a special clinic in Mexico where he could receive the 'wonder drug', laetrile (vitamin B_{17}). They also discussed the possibility of sending him to a cancer specialist working in New Zealand. They had mentioned this plan to the doctors in the outpatients' clinic and were berated angrily for contemplating 'such nonsense'.

My inexperience was now apparent and I found this problem threatening; I asked them to give me two days and then I would contact them. The phone bill soared as I contacted experts around the country. I then informed the family that they should save their money because the results of treatment for cerebral tumours were poor. However, I told them that Neil could acquire the therapeutic dose of vitamin B_{17} by ingesting 15–20 apricot kernels each day. They all seemed satisfied by this compromise and so poor Neil chewed the bitter kernels every day.

I agreed to make home visits each week to encourage him and his wife with positive thinking and support. To our amazement, instead of arranging a funeral six months later, we were arranging his driver's licence, an easy job and even Australian rules football. In fact, we were wondering if the tumour had been cured, but eight years later he started to have convulsions again, deteriorated gradually and died at the age of 31, leaving a wife, three children and happy memories of at least seven years of good health after the operation.

DISCUSSION AND LESSONS LEARNED

- The importance of early diagnosis of malignant disease is obvious, but such a diagnosis is not always easy in a busy general practice where the symptoms usually represent a more common disease. It is questionable whether early diagnosis leads to a better outcome for some malignancies; at least it is good for our professional image and may prevent patients from getting into the clutches of charlatans and the non-evidence-based alternative practitioners.
- The intensity of the feelings of grieving relatives and friends cannot be underestimated. Our patients do get angry and aggressive and such emotion is not always obvious. Our counselling and management plan should take this into account.
- It is a mistake to prognosticate about life expectancy.
- It is also a mistake to be dogmatic and uncompromising with patients when they seek advice about other methods of treatment. It is important to offer sympathy and guidance and provide hope whenever possible.
- Remember the old Persian proverb: 'You cannot recall the spoken word, the spent arrow or the lost opportunity'.

A cruel world

Glimpses of a cruel world

The local Health Officer met me outside the house. 'She's a widow living alone . . . a recluse . . . she's boarded up all the windows and locked herself in . . . hasn't paid gas, electricity or water bills for months and so all those services have been stopped . . . the folk next door sell her water for 50 cents a bucket,' he paused. 'Bit of a health hazard now.'

He produced a key and a powerful torch and led the way. Inside it was as dark as a tomb. He forced the shutters open and suddenly daylight flooded into the living room, which presented an extraordinary sight. Furniture was piled and stacked so that you could barely move, with new bird cages and an ironing board propped against a grand piano. And everywhere giant black cobwebs. 'She's a compulsive spender . . . here she comes.'

A fantastic sight met our eyes. Two very white human legs wriggled in mid-air in the beam of his torch. Then the feet found their way to the floor. An adult torso now started to worm its way backwards out of the waist-high tunnel. Eventually a woman dressed in black stood up. 'Good afternoon,' she said, in an exquisitely modulated English voice.

'Good afternoon, Mrs Digby,' said my companion. 'She lives down there,' he said. He shone the torch down the tunnel, which proved to be constructed of furniture and roughly floored with cushions. 'There's a kitchen at the far end,' and I could see a mongrel-looking dog tethered to the gas stove.

'But how . . .' I began.

'There's a back door leading to the yard,' he said. 'They both use it!'

'And how are you, Mrs Digby?'

'If I'd known you were coming I'd have had the kettle on,' she said demurely.

'She's not pregnant, Doctor'

She lay back wanly against the pillows, a white-faced married woman aged 30. I was doing a short-term stint at a small town hospital. She admitted to few symptoms.

'I just feel exhausted,' she murmured softly. She was breathing quickly, but heart and lungs seemed normal to my examination.

'I'll just check your tummy,' I said.

Some instinct made me lift the sheet. Between her legs was a severed umbilical cord.

'You've just had a baby,' I announced naively.

'Oh no, Doctor,' she replied. 'I'm not pregnant'. Further questioning elicited further denials.

Her husband would have been in his 40s, and looked grey and tired. 'Oh no, Doctor, she's not pregnant,' he maintained. And then added, by way of oblique explanation, 'I work nights, you see, and she's on days.'

'Has she perhaps been in another hospital?' My tone must have sounded dumbfounded.

'No—she's just been at home with me.'

The woman police constable seated at the bedside looked incongruous in the little hospital ward. At home, in a suitcase, the bodies of twin boys had been found, their heads showing signs of severe contusion where they had struck the tiled floor of the bathroom.

I attended the post-mortem on the babies, done by a well-known forensic pathologist. 'One of the more heart-rending crimes, I always think,' he said. 'Infanticide—and you wonder why it isn't commoner than it is.'

Trying to catch the bus

I was on casualty duty in the same hospital. An elderly man had just walked in.

'I was just trying to catch the bus,' he said forlornly. He held out a hand. At first glance the thumb appeared to have been almost severed. In fact some skin and, mercifully, a core of tendon and connective tissue were still holding it on. This was well before the days of microsurgery. As I bent over to infiltrate, I noticed that his pain responses seemed satisfactorily dulled. He had a bland, facile grin on his face, and it was the face of a man in his late 60s.

'I was running behind and tried to jump on,' he explained. As I worked on I noticed that he seemed insensitive to pain, even in areas where I had not injected local. I had been qualified for all of eight weeks, and my mind wrestled with a diagnosis. I finished my needle-work and stood up.

'I want you to come back tomorrow for a fresh dressing,' I said, putting what I hoped was a friendly reassuring hand on his left upper arm as I did so. To my dismay his left humerus 'clunked' with an extraordinary display of crepitus and was clearly broken. Yet he did not even wince!

'I think you'd better sit down again,' I said. I wrote a letter referring him to the nearest public hospital. An ambulance could take him at once.

A further emergency had just come in, and Sister was tugging at my arm. I ended my letter with the words '. . . I have not checked his femurs'.

You've guessed it. He had a fractured femur as well. And the cause of his anaesthesia? I never discovered.

DISCUSSION AND LESSONS LEARNED

Although we lead varied lives, there are certainly moments when we seem to be caught up in a dull routine. Then the veil may suddenly lift and we are face-to-face with a startling glimpse of a cruel world normally beyond our ken, in which ordinary folk are battling with mental confusion, grievous personal loss, pain and deprivation. And they need our respect and understanding as much as, if not more than, the conventionally ill.

The sting of death: chilling visits

Visit 1

'For God's sake, Doctor, can you come immediately to Jack's place? It's Bert calling. Please come quick—it's a matter of life and death,' was the dramatic phone call that interrupted my morning surgery. The urgency and drama from Jack's brother was so compelling that I excused myself with apologies to the patients in the waiting room (a common event in a country practice) and sped towards Jack's humble shack in the bush some 18 km away. Jack was a 58-year-old bachelor, who led a virtual hermit's existence tending his considerable variety of animals.

My heart sank as my speeding car momentarily lost control, when I rounded a sharp bend with poor camber on the winding road to his shack in the hills. I then recalled my father's advice that 'a smashed-up doctor would be more than useless to a dying patient' and travelled at a more realistic speed.

When I pulled up by the shack in a cloud of dust I was greeted by a pack of excited dogs and Bert, who said, 'It's not pretty, Doc'. I then realised that I had been monumentally misled. Poor old Jack's corpse was beyond resuscitation. He had been dead at least 10 days and his decaying flesh was being eaten by his starving dogs.

Visit 2

'Doctor, could you come down and help us. There's an elderly lady who's really sick and can't wake up or something. She's with an elderly citizens group from Melbourne.' This was the urgent call from the ranger in charge of a recreational park, which was a popular day picnic spot for city people. 'Hypoglycaemic,' I thought.

It took me 20 minutes to reach the park where the scene that greeted me was quite extraordinary. An elderly lady sat alone in a folding chair as though asleep in the middle of an area with about three hundred people standing back in a circle at least 30 m from her (Figure 8.1). I wondered if an explosive device was on her person, but the poor dear was sleeping peacefully and permanently. As I approached her the mass closely followed me, 'We don't know her—she has no friends or relatives with her. Is she going to be

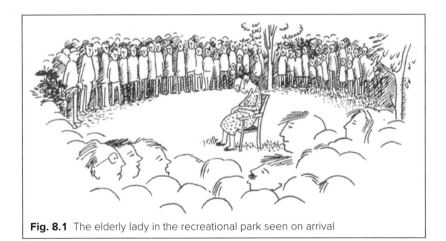

Fig. 8.1 The elderly lady in the recreational park seen on arrival

all right?' Guess who knew she was dead but was denying it? And guess who spent the next two hours of his precious time organising the unhappy formalities? I often reflect that in real life I would have loved to have known her and spoken with her.

Visit 3

On another occasion I received an urgent call from a farmhouse by the local dam, a huge expanse of water that provided water for part of the metropolitan area and also for local consumption. The caller said that there was a fisherman who was extremely sick and unable to be moved, and that his friend needed a doctor urgently. As there was no local ambulance stationed in our town I travelled to the area, whereupon I was led on a long and arduous snake-infested trek that only fisherfolk seemed prepared to undertake. Ninety minutes later I reached a very dead person, who had died suddenly from a myocardial infarction doing what he loved best. His companion said, 'I feared the worst but you never know.'

Visit 4

Sweet, gentle, old Mrs C rang me at 6.15 am to request a home visit because her husband George seemed so cold in bed and would not rouse. Sensing the worst, I sped to the neat homely abode where a rather composed and matter-of-fact lady led me to George, who had obviously been dead for several hours. I asked her to wait in the kitchen as I went through the motions of resuscitation for five minutes and then went out to solemnly inform her that 'I couldn't save him—I think he must have stopped breathing just as you noticed him cold'. 'I thought it was too late', came the reply.

DISCUSSIONS AND LESSONS LEARNED

- Coping with death from one's own viewpoint and that of the bereaved friends and relatives is never easy and keeps us humble as we face our own mortality and the limitations of our healing art. In one way death represents professional failure, yet our greatest failure is not providing appropriate care, responsibility and counselling for the family in crisis. The last is an ever-present challenge.

- Lay people may find it hard to recognise death and then cope with it rationally. It paralyses so many. While seeming to deny its reality they depend so much on their doctor to 'come to the rescue'. In country practice the general practitioner seems to be the focal point—not the police or the clergy. We have to be prepared for this responsibility.
- Dropping everything and racing to the scene of 'crisis' can be a time-consuming and even dangerous procedure. It pays to be ever alert when taking the phone call to extract sufficient information from the distressed caller to get the visit into perspective. It is advisable to take the message directly rather than responding to a 'please attend' by one's receptionist or other party.
- It is vital to be sensitive to the feelings and responses of loved ones so that the bereavement reaction is softened as much as possible. Alleviating their guilt is an important consideration even if it means 'playing games' as with Mrs C. For example, living with the realisation of sleeping through the night alongside a dead loved one can be a terrible burden to carry. Honesty and open disclosure are important but there are times when we give more when we give less information (see Dr David Korones' wonderful article 'The Long Ride Home', *NEJM,* 2017).
- It is also vital to explain to relatives exactly how and why their loved one died: the conducting of an autopsy can certainly provide the basis for a proper explanation.

Haunting images of lifeless children

The saddest and most haunting memories of my professional career are the deaths of children, which seem to be like beautiful buds of a flower snapped off so prematurely and cruelly. The following experiences encountered while working in the emergency department of the Royal Children's Hospital are self-explanatory.

- The 18-month-old daughter of a busy medical family arrived one evening with severe burns to 80 per cent of her body, caused by being placed in a bath of piping hot water by her 9-year-old sister who had the task of bathing her. Her agony was eventually ended by her death in hospital.
- DOAs (dead on arrival) of 2-year-olds found floating in the backyard swimming pool and others crushed by their parents' car in the driveways of their homes were so distressing, especially for the parents. I can never forget the case of a 3-week-old baby in a carrying basket who was run over by the mother in a car park as she reversed the car over the basket, after absent mindedly forgetting to place the basket in the car when she loaded shopping items into the car boot.
- A 3-year-old died from injuries received from falling off the roof of a house after climbing a ladder left against the house.
- Epiglottitis (thankfully rare now with Hib immunisation), croup, asthma: deaths from these lethal respiratory problems seemed commonplace. In one month I encountered four DOAs from epiglottitis, with one child arriving with a piece of tubing from a Littmann's stethoscope acting as a tracheostomy, which was bravely inserted by a general practitioner who accompanied the child in the ambulance.
- Acute gastroenteritis in infants: now there's a problem that is real and often underestimated. In some instances death or severe illness occurred from inappropriate advice, including giving saltwater or copious amounts of lemonade to the infants to drink.

DISCUSSION AND LESSONS LEARNED

- The importance of giving advice to parents about child accident prevention in the home was obvious and eventually became an obsession. An educational sheet for all new parents was devised. Such advice included the following:
  - put all spray cleaners, kerosene, pesticides, rat poison and so on out of children's reach

-   don't use tablecloths with toddlers around
-   run cold water before hot into children's baths
-   get rid of plastic covers; don't leave them lying around
-   don't leave ladders around and take special care when mowing lawns
-   in a pool, 5 cm of water is sufficient to drown a toddler
-   place your child in the car first and then walk right around the car before reversing down the drive. All children should be placed in an approved child restraint even to be driven just around the corner.

- Upon commencing country general practice, I made the provision of resuscitation equipment for children a priority. The resuscitation kit included paediatric endotracheal tubes with introducers, paediatric tracheostomy tubes, butterfly needles, intravenous cutdown equipment and so on. We purchased the latest aids for asthma including pumps, nebulisers and the latest delivery systems, which were loaned to families of asthmatics. We commenced education classes in prevention and first aid, and these became a popular and regular feature in our community. The community awareness of preventive strategies for common causes of morbidity and mortality made the effort extremely rewarding.

- In 10 years of private practice, during which I cared for 2700 patients, I encountered only two childhood deaths: a 2-year-old with Hand–Schüller–Christian disease and a 13-year-old who sustained head injuries following a fall onto a hurdle rail while horse riding (her helmet was not secured and it fell off as she was thrown from the horse). Perhaps our strategy was very successful, or we were lucky, or both. However, it was immensely satisfying to have no deaths from respiratory diseases.

Where there's a will . . .

After many years with dementia and immobility Bill's death came as no surprise. What did come as a surprise was a letter from a lawyer acting on behalf of Bill's son to his GP. The lawyer wanted a medico-legal report from the GP about Bill's testamentary capacity two years before his death.

Apparently Bill had made a new will at this time which had left all of his assets to his paid carer and nothing to his four children.

DISCUSSION AND LESSONS LEARNED

- Testamentary capacity is a specific legal concept which refers to the ability of a person to make a will. The required capacity will vary with the complexity of the will and potential claimants involved.
- The legal test is surprisingly old—found in the English 1870 case of *Banks v Goodfellow* and still relied on by lawyers today. The case involved the writer of a will who had delusions—but were the delusions enough to invalidate his will? The court concluded they were not and that the will was valid.
- The legal test for determining if an individual possesses sufficient capacity to make a will requires the person to:
    - understand the nature of making a will and its effects
    - understand the extent of the assets they are bequeathing
    - comprehend and appreciate the (moral) claims to which they must give effect
    - not be affected by a disorder of the mind that 'shall poison his affections, pervert his sense of right, or prevent the exercise of his natural faculties'.

Going up in smoke

Even though a will can be disputed after a person's death, it's probably a better outcome than having no will at all.

I had one cranky, old wealthy matriarch who didn't like her children and said to me, 'They are not going to get my money (wads of notes and bonds). Doctor, I will hide them in my old stove' (huge metal bomb that it was). Soon after she died, her son came in upset that they couldn't find mum's money. I didn't reveal her secret. Then he said, 'We had this huge burn up in the old stove and fire place.' Holy smoke!

Chapter 9

The concealment syndrome

The ticket of entry

Margot

'Doctor, it's Margot. I think I've got the shingles again: there's another rash on my right leg. What do you think?'

'I think we'd better take a look. Come in later this afternoon.'

Margot arrived and there were a few spots on the leg previously affected by shingles, but they were not typical of her recent virus: they were itchy rather than painful.

'It's certainly not shingles. How do you feel generally?'

'I feel terrible,' she said and then burst into tears.

The rash had been a 'ticket of entry'.

Margot then explained how tense, irritable and depressed she had been since her husband had retired. Jack, under pressure from his wife, had chosen early retirement at 60, despite excellent physical and mental health. It was thought that now the family had grown up there would be time for them to do things together. The reality was quite different. 'He's there all the time; keeps getting under my feet. I love him so much and yet I'm unpleasant to him. I feel that because he's at home I've been demoted from captain to lieutenant.' The consultation went on in this vein for a long time.

I first heard the expression 'ticket of entry' from my partner, Geoff Ryan, Foundation Professor of Community Practice at the University of Queensland. He had coined the phrase during a discussion about the ways patients would conceal their reasons for seeking advice. Hesitation to broach the subject immediately could be due to many factors: guilt and embarrassment, as in Margot's case; fear of the unknown (or known); inability to discuss personal matters easily; or apparent loss of face.

Harry

Harry was a 35-year-old strong, healthy man who earned his living by laying concrete and prided himself on his physique and strength of character.

'It's this elbow again, Doctor. I think I'll need the injection after all; I can't do my job properly.'

I examined, concurred and gave the injection of steroid.

'You knew I was a professional marksman?' said Harry. I had to confess that I did not. 'I'm having terrible trouble with palpitations before the big events: puts me right off. Can you do anything to help?'

I sat down to tackle the real reason for the consultation: his 'macho image' had been eroded. Fear is a common reason for use of the 'ticket'.

Mrs M

Mrs M was a woman in her 40s who kept good health and was only an occasional patient. I had not seen her for some time.

'I'm due for my Pap smear.'

After checking her medical records to confirm her last result I followed the routine procedure. I asked if she did regular breast self-examination. She replied, 'I came here today because there's a lump in my right breast.' There was.

Gerry

Gerry, a large, A-grade squash player in his mid-30s, was mildly hypertensive and overweight. He appeared one day, concerned about his weight and its effect on his knees and ankles. We discussed it fully.

'Jenny has been complaining.' I waited for him to elaborate on his wife's complaint. 'I can't maintain an erection.' Embarrassment and 'macho loss' were evident once more.

DISCUSSION AND LESSONS LEARNED

- These are four examples of a common phenomenon in general practice. In my experience this delay in getting to the point occurs when the problem is personal: marital upset, breakdown of a relationship and, most often, the embarrassment of discussing a problem of a sexual nature.
- The message for the general practitioner is to be patient during the consultation. The apparent reason for presentation might be a mask that will be raised eventually to reveal the true face. People can find it difficult to open up to their doctor immediately, no matter how comforting or relaxed we think we are.
- We must try to discipline ourselves against irritation when, having solved what seems to be the obvious problem, we find it is only a 'ticket of entry'.

The concealment enigma: why is it so?

> **Duke:** And what's her history?
> **Viola:** A blank, my Lord: She never told her love, But let concealment, like a worm i' the bud, Feed on her damask cheek: she pin'd in thought; And, with a green and yellow melancholy, She sat, like patience on a monument, Smiling at grief.

William Shakespeare, *Twelfth Night*, Act II, Scene IV

Mrs A

Mrs A, a 66-year-old woman, sat on the edge of the bed, deathly pale, wet with cold perspiration, obviously in extreme distress. The pain described was classic: retrosternal, crushing and radiating down the left arm. She had a long history of hypertension with ischaemic heart disease. This night her blood pressure was very low, the tachycardia rapid but regular, and the pain supreme. A definite myocardial infarct. Despite the distress she was reluctant to bare her chest. The reason was soon evident. In the upper outer quadrant of the left breast was a hard ulcerated carcinoma of the breast, which had been there for well over a year. (Refer to Figure 9.1, centre insert page 5.) She had told no one, not even her husband.

Mrs Y

Mrs Y always accompanied her husband on his routine visits: she literally led him by the hand. He had a long history of peripheral vascular disease and controlled cardiac arrhythmia. Arthur—a pleasant, chatty, ingenuous man—needed looking after. His wife always wore a headscarf. One day with some embarrassment she removed it. The right ear was absent—replaced by an invading basal cell carcinoma. Though it had been present for at least 18 months no one had been informed. Her husband had not noticed it.

Mr B

I was introduced to Mr B by his wife, who said there was something wrong with his upper lip. I looked at what I thought was an untreated harelip and cleft palate in a small, thin, aggressive 61-year-old who did not like doctors. He had otherwise been in perfect health and obviously thought his lip would get better if ignored. His wife, risking his displeasure, had taken her courage in both hands and called me. A rodent ulcer had eroded half his upper lip through to the nasal septum, giving the harelip appearance.

Mrs G

Mrs G, a lady of 54 years of age, was pale, thin and already cachectic. She sat up weakly in bed in a pink dressing gown while her husband stood guiltily in the background. The air in the bedroom smelt of putrefaction. In tears she slipped off the dressing gown to reveal the fungating remnant of her left breast. Axillary lymph glands were easily palpable and a pleural effusion present, yet she had told no one. Her husband said he did not know about it. In the presence of such obvious illness and deathly odour, how could it have been missed?

How can this possibly happen?

Those of us who have been in general practice for any length of time have seen such cases and never fail to be surprised or even horrified by them.

They are good examples of the phenomenon of concealment. It commonly but not always occurs in happily married older people when the bloom of youth and sexual communication have gone.

Why do these people suffer in silence? Fear of what is believed to be inevitable? Protection of the beloved spouse? Dismissal as an unacceptable occurrence? A fatalistic philosophy? In many instances it is not lack of intellect, because these patients cover the full spectrum of intelligence. Whatever the reason it is a heartbreaking and sickening experience for the doctor who is unfortunate to be present at the unveiling; his or her presence like a prophet of doom.

And what became of these victims of concealment?

The lady who had the infarct while concealing her breast is still alive but her cardiac state is critical. We are all hoping this will solve the problem of other medical decisions.

The protective lady who led her husband by the hand is now a widow: her husband had a fatal heart attack. She had the ear remnant and supporting tissue removed, now wears her hair long and spurns an expensive artificial ear.

The man with the upper lip neoplasm is hale, hearty and as aggressive as ever. A series of constructive repair procedures over many months looks like a successful repair of an old harelip.

And the lady with the ulcerating, fungating breast neoplasm? She suffered a painful, emaciating, lingering death. I continued to see her husband regularly; he never mentioned her again.

DISCUSSION AND LESSONS LEARNED

- Every doctor should be aware that some people, for a variety of reasons, conceal their illnesses. The competent doctor, alert for signs of this, can make the opening for which the patient is waiting.
- This requires at all times the exercise of sensitivity, understanding and tact. Sometimes a doctor will develop a 'sixth sense' of perception that the patient's presenting symptoms are not those that are most worrying him or her, or in most need of attention.

Fitting the drug abuse jigsaw together

Case 1

Michelle G, a 14-year-old schoolgirl, presented with colicky abdominal pain of two months' duration. Apart from some anorexia and nausea there were no associated symptoms, such as a change in bowel habits or evidence of menstruation-related pain. She had visited a naturopath who said it was irritable bowel and provided dietary advice plus some medicine. In taking the history I asked casually, 'How many cigarettes do you smoke each day?' The furtive glance between mother and daughter was highly significant. Before she had time to deny it I asked, 'Six, ten or twenty?' 'Just a few', came the sheepish reply.

I informed her surprised mother, 'Michelle has the problem of 'schoolgirl's colic'—a common problem in those starting smoking cigarettes. Nicotine is a drug and can cause these physiological effects, which soon settle but it's best to quit now.' They went home with advice and handouts on quitting smoking.

Case 2

Peter S, aged 23, presented because he was feeling flat and listless. His parents who accompanied him claimed he 'wasn't himself'—he was bored, lazy, apathetic and did not care about his work on the farm. He would not get out of bed to milk the cows and had been in trouble with motor accidents, and law and disorder.

Peter seemed unwell, apathetic and uninterested in the consultation. While taking a history I gained the impression that he had mental health problems although he denied any symptoms. 'How much pot, grass or dope are you smoking, Peter?'

'Yeah—quite a bit—everyone's smoking the stuff.' His parents had no idea that he was smoking it.

Case 3

Mandy E, a 16-year-old schoolgirl was being 'nursed' at home for suspected gastroenteritis. I was asked to visit her because she was very sick and her abdominal pain becoming more intense. 'Pelvic appendicitis,' I thought en route to the humble home in a small township. Her mother claimed, 'She's been acting strange, has twitches in her muscles and is yawning a lot today.' She had a two-day history of nausea, running eyes and nose, colicky abdominal pain and diarrhoea. Physical examination was normal.

I was aware that heroin had been introduced into the area. Mandy was an obvious case of heroin withdrawal.

Case 4

Hal J, a 42-year-old actor, came to see me because he had collapsed late one evening. 'He's been working his butt off and is physically and mentally exhausted,' claimed a friend who brought in the fidgety, sweating and floppy patient. His blood pressure was 180/110 and his pulse 102. I performed an ECG, which showed runs of ventricular premature beats. I admitted him to hospital where he became very languid, irritable and aggressive (at times), and ground his teeth incessantly. After 24 hours he became paranoid and apparently psychotic, with disorganised thinking.

It was obvious that he was having a withdrawal from a stimulant drug (perhaps amphetamines). I asked him and his associates about this possibility and determined that he was taking 'crack'—the stronger alkaloid derivative of cocaine.

DISCUSSION AND LESSONS LEARNED

- All these cases illustrate the wide variety of manifestations of substance abuse, each representing a diagnostic conundrum. Cocaine is a rather overpowering drug; no less dangerous is our most serious drug problem—nicotine abuse.
- We have to suspect drug abuse, especially in teenagers and those who may be exposed to the drug scene presenting with poor health, unusual symptoms, and changes in personality and school performance. An apparent psychotic episode may also be a strong pointer to abuse of illicit drugs.

Distracted by mother's presence

Meredith was a 23-year-old lawyer who presented to our practice with
a gastrointestinal disturbance. She was seen by the GP registrar and was
accompanied by her mother who was a rather severe and clinging personality.
She would give the history in tandem with her daughter who did look
somewhat pale and distracted.

Meredith had a past history of migraine and anorexia nervosa. She had
been quite well in the previous few years while she completed her law degree
and had attended the practice for prescriptions of the oral contraceptive pill.

Her presenting complaint was anorexia and nausea with mild left colicky
abdominal pain. She had loose bowel actions and had vomited three times
in the past 12 hours. On examination her vital signs were pulse 64/min,
BP 100/65, temperature 36.7 °C, respiratory rate 14/min. On abdominal
examination there was mild tenderness in the left flank and left iliac fossa
while the rectal examination was normal.

I agreed with my colleague that the diagnosis was rather obscure but that
a working diagnosis of gastroenteritis was appropriate. She was sent home
with the advice to ring us at the surgery if there were any further problems.

Mother rang the next day to say that she was worried about Meredith
because of increased colicky pain and discoloured urine. I went on a home
visit and found the patient looking worse than the previous day and certainly
wan and depressed. Mother remained in the thick of the process offering her
own differential diagnoses. The urine specimen contained blood and she now
had dysuria and I wondered about possible acute pyelonephritis although she
was afebrile.

I organised for her to attend a colleague at a nearby emergency facility for
investigations including FBE, ESR, MCU and renal ultrasound. The FBE was
normal (including platelets), ESR 45 and the ultrasound revealed obstruction
of the left renal pelvis probably due to blood clot. An INR ordered by my
astute colleague was 7.0. Strange. So a more detailed history was taken.

Would you believe Meredith had been feeling depressed to the point she
felt suicidal? She started to ingest 'Ratsak', which she understood would be
an effective poison. However, after a few days nothing much was happening

apart from the sick feelings and she now felt 'extremely stupid' about her actions and believed that if she kept quiet then the substance would dissipate and no one would need to know.

DISCUSSION AND LESSONS LEARNED

- Once again the importance of a good family history is highlighted.
- Be somewhat sceptical especially if the situation seems unusual and don't assume that nice people don't do weird things.
- If you sense that it is appropriate, see the patient alone if possible. It may be necessary to diplomatically ask another person, relative or friend, to leave the room.
- Ask the patient what they consider 'is their real problem'.
- Always believe and take cognisance of a mother's concern.

Paper-clip problems

How often have we been 'caught out' by the paper-clip trap whereby a loose A4 page gets inadvertently attached to the back of an unrelated document when it is bound by a paper clip? A vain search for the document may follow. All may be revealed when the lost document is found in a week, a month or even a year's time—or never!

Mrs CS, a 43-year-old lawyer, received a paper copy of her Pap smear result together with the vaginal swab results of another patient. They were posted out from our practice following the sequence of *GP→practice nurse→receptionist→patient.*

Mrs CS phoned to express her displeasure at this clanger and organised to return the report to the practice for shredding according to confidentiality protocol. The error occurred when the reception staff clipped the results of the two different patients together. The error was not detected by the doctor's checks, the computer or by the reception staff printing the address stickers. A letter of apology to both patients followed and the practice reviewed its policy of handling paper results.

DISCUSSION AND LESSONS LEARNED

- Although this incident did not compromise patient health it was unprofessional, embarrassing and potentially litigious.
- In our practice paper clips are no longer used for the collation of patients' results or reports.
- Other remedial strategies include doctors and practice nurses carefully scrutinising every paper report, and reception staff checking the content of all envelopes to be posted prior to sealing them.
- The widespread use of electronic health records now means there is a risk of large-scale breaches of patient confidentiality, such as when a database containing medical records is hacked. Under the Notifiable Data Breaches legislation, if an eligible data breach occurs in your practice, you are required to notify any individuals at risk of serious harm and also the Office of the Australian Information Commissioner.

Chapter 10

Families in conflict

Throwing baby out with the bathwater

Wendy, aged 26, was the self-possessed, dynamic theatre nurse of a nearby hospital who was married to a logging contractor. She was delighted with her first child delivered under our care. Over subsequent weeks she presented for help and advice at least weekly with her baby boy. There was some uncharacteristic irritation when we advised against circumcision. However, knowing her personality, I reassured her (and myself) that she would cope just fine.

Her husband rang me to say that he was concerned about Wendy because she had 'lost interest in him, the household and sex', among other things. She was also 'bitchy and flying off the handle easily'. When I next saw Wendy, I discussed many of her problems and said I thought she had postpartum depression and should take medication in addition to counselling and support from myself. She dismissed her problems as simple 'postnatal blues' and said that she did not need, nor would she take any medication.

Diagnosis and outcome

One week later Geoff rang to request a house call. When I arrived I found Wendy slumped on the kitchen table weeping while Geoff was holding the baby. 'I came in to find her trying to drown the baby, and then she was going to slash her wrists,' he said.

'I'm just a failure as a mother and a wife. Everyone thinks I'm hopeless. I am hopeless,' whimpered Wendy.

Wendy eventually responded to support, amitriptyline and electroconvulsive therapy. It took about 12 months for her to return to her normal, effervescent, coping self.

A classic case of postnatal depression had emerged under our noses and we were fortunate not to be answerable to a case of infanticide and suicide.

DISCUSSION AND LESSONS LEARNED

- Depression, including postnatal depression, is potentially a deadly problem. Apart from the possibility of suicide, it can cause havoc in the home. I have encountered broken marriages and strained marriages through one of the partners being depressed.
- Depression is a very real illness that affects the entire mind and body. It seriously dampens the five basic activities of humans, namely activity, sex, sleep, appetite and the ability to cope with life. Place this into a household and the 'rotten apple' effect can take over with relationships seriously affected.
- We have a tendency to continue to treat people as we normally know them and tend to deny that they are mentally ill or rationalise that any deviant behaviour is but a passing phase. Experience has shown that doctors cannot take anything for granted with psychiatric illness, especially depressive illness.
- Subsequent to this experience I have always searched for evidence of depression early in the postpartum phase and, if present, treated it aggressively.

Piggy in the middle

At times it can be difficult in general practice to avoid becoming embroiled in the acrimony between separated parents. The key goal in this situation is to prevent you and your practice from getting caught up in a dispute between the parents, while continuing to provide medical care and act in the best interests of the child.

The father of a 5-year-old patient saw the GP registrar on a Saturday morning to obtain a prescription for an EpiPen Jr® for his son. The father said he needed an EpiPen® when he had his son on weekend access visits, in view of the patient's severe peanut allergy. The GP printed a prescription for the child and gave it to the father.

A few weeks later, the GP received a letter of complaint from the patient's mother. The letter stated her ex-husband had sent her a copy of the prescription, 'taunting' her with the fact that he now knew her address. She had a Violence Restraining Order against the father which prohibited him from making any contact with her. The prescription the GP had given to the father included the mother's address. Unfortunately, there was no information in the child's medical records to alert the GP to this situation.

DISCUSSION AND LESSONS LEARNED

- In general terms, either parent of a young child can obtain a copy of their child's medical records, or information about their health care. However, it is worth being wary of a request for access to medical records or information about a child where the parents are separated or divorced.
- Before providing a parent with medical records or information about their child, carefully review the information to ensure it does not contain information relating to another person.
- If you are unsure how to proceed, it's worth seeking advice—you may be able to avoid becoming 'piggy in the middle' of a dispute that should not involve you or your practice.

Lame duck survival

Oh, your precious lame ducks.

John Galsworthy, *The Man of Property*, Part 2, Ch. 12

All of us in general practice become familiar with the situation that lends itself to the label 'lame duck survival'. Typically, two people are involved;

perhaps they are sisters who have not married and live together, or are a married couple without children. When one member becomes permanently ill or disabled the balance of the partnership often alters: the healthy partner takes on the role of caretaker, manager and controller; the other becomes totally dependent. This is not the catastrophe one might imagine; the once dependent partner—the 'lame duck'—survives, often coping remarkably well.

Mrs C's lame ducks

Mrs C's case illustrates an extreme example: she became responsible for a whole flock of 'lame ducks'.

Married at an early age and against the wishes of her family, Mrs C strictly and carefully raised four healthy children (two boys and two girls). Gradually it became apparent to her that the attractive young man she married was becoming ineffectual and difficult, dependent yet aggressive; his behaviour was strange and incomprehensible. Eventually he became psychotic and was diagnosed as a chronic schizophrenic.

Mrs C's two daughters married (at a relatively early age, as their mother had done) and each had two children. For some reason these offspring (all male) became difficult and 'hyperactive'; Mrs C agreed to take a large share of the burden of minding her grandsons. This she did in addition to taking on a job as a chef's assistant (to prop up their ailing family finances) and looking after her psychologically disabled husband.

Mrs C had a strong personality indeed, but worse was to follow. Her eldest son, handsome and bright, refused tertiary education and chose apprenticeship to a bricklayer. Without warning he became severely depressed and suicidal and, despite hospitalisation, electroconvulsive therapy and antidepressant medication, took a rifle from his treasured gun collection and shot himself. As a suicide attempt it was unsuccessful but it destroyed his eyesight. Discharged from medical care, he went home to the care of his mother.

By now Mrs C's parents were old, infirm and becoming totally dependent. Being their only daughter, Mrs C was expected to look after them; this she did.

The catastrophe

Eventually the death of Mrs C's aged mother (from renal failure) alleviated her caretaker load a little. Then one morning, totally unexpectedly, the dominant and apparently indestructible Mrs C was found dead in bed. Her family was stunned; even as he administered the last rites, the parish priest expected her eyes to open at any moment.

The consequences

Mrs C's father was admitted quickly to a nursing home. Her two daughters and their difficult sons matured remarkably quickly. The indifferent Mr C sold the family home and, with his blind son, moved into a town house where he lived in a zombie-like state with tardive dyskinesia and monthly phenothiazine injections. Amazingly, Mrs C's son began to function relatively well: perhaps he assumed a type of caretaker role? (Mrs C's youngest son, her fourth child, had managed to escape the family turmoil. Although dependent on his mother, he matured through a trade apprenticeship and marriage and is well.)

DISCUSSION AND LESSONS LEARNED

It is difficult for a general practitioner to intervene in the problems of such a family but no person should be allowed to take on, alone, that breadth of responsibility. Dare we try to interfere?

The hubris syndrome

Tom was a dashing young man-about-town who was greatly admired for his various skills, especially as a sporting hero. He was an outstanding Australian Rules football player and a gifted cricketer and golfer. In addition he was a highly paid coach of a leading football team. He was tall, dark and handsome and also extremely charming, which led to his popularity—especially with women. He would consult me regularly because of various musculoskeletal complaints and I did detect a certain arrogance, as though he knew better than health professionals and boasted about his great powers of healing.

Tom was married with two children. As he moved into his 30s family problems started surfacing, including complaints from his wife, who was experiencing anxiety about Tom's behaviour. He had become inattentive, stayed out late partying and was bullying her and the children. There was talk that he was considering running for selection as a parliamentary candidate. On one occasion she confided that she believed the problem was related to the fact that he 'was up himself'. I knew what she was talking about. His philandering, exaggerated self-importance and overwhelming self-confidence were also starting to affect other families and marriages. One night he was admitted to the emergency room with injuries from an assault from the partner of a woman Tom had allegedly become involved with. Eventually his marriage broke down as his wife could not cope with the humiliation of her situation. We had to provide considerable support and counselling for this disturbed albeit gifted man.

DISCUSSION AND LESSONS LEARNED

- Tom is an example of the hubris syndrome, which was aptly named by (Dr) Lord David Owen as he identified George Bush, Tony Blair and Margaret Thatcher as prime examples in his books *The Hubris Syndrome* and *In Sickness and in Power* (Owen, 2007; 2008). Not surprisingly he listed Adolf Hitler and his followers as classic (and extreme) cases. The *Oxford Dictionary* defines 'hubris' as 'arrogant pride and excessive self-confidence leading to insolence and possible self destruction (nemesis)'.

- We can identify certain notable sporting identities, actors, musicians, politicians and others who exhibit the syndrome. It appears that those affected harbour a narcissistic personality disorder which may be innate or latent (precipitated by fame and/or power). Some psychiatrists consider that the syndrome could also be a manifestation of bipolar disorder. The person in question is not easy to manage, nor are the disrupted relationships, but it's helpful for family doctors to be aware of the syndrome and its effect on family and community health.

Abdominal pain beyond belief

Billy was one of those patients who haunts every practice. Completely self-indulgent and doctor-dependent, he was reliant on every drug that would help blot out reality: alcohol, morphine, amphetamines and (in those days) Relaxa-tabs. His medical records carried the somewhat elitist diagnosis of Munchausen syndrome—an unfortunate label that eventually was to affect his management adversely.

Aged 38, Billy was an almost comical-looking man of short, obese stature, who tended to communicate with a staccato of almost inaudible grunts (Figure 11.1). Nevertheless, there was something appealing about this harmless roly-poly Dickensian character.

He would present with a dramatic episode of abdominal pain (invariably in the evening) at our surgery or the emergency department of the teaching hospital, where he virtually had a mortgage on a surgical bed following an appendicectomy and a cholecystectomy. He appeared to be a world authority on the symptoms and signs of acute pancreatitis.

We were convinced that the strategy of treating his abdominal pain in hospital with a nasogastric milk drip was proving effective because his visits were now infrequent. Billy was, however, seeking comfort from his Relaxa-tabs despite many visits to drug treatment centres.

I will never forget the day when Billy presented in the morning complaining of the eternal abdominal pain: 'It's the worst gut-ache I've ever had, Doc'. As he sat in front of me, like a melancholy bullfrog, my imagination drifted fiendishly and most unprofessionally to the scenarios of Ian Fleming's novels in which trapdoors under chairs lead to tanks of sharks, crocodiles or (best of all) piranha fish. Eventually poor Billy was dispatched, unhappily clutching a prescription for an antacid.

I was not exactly overjoyed when he reappeared at 11 pm claiming he had been treated rudely at the hospital emergency department. Yet, for once in his life, Billy looked genuinely ill. Examination of his abdomen revealed more than his usual guarding and tenderness: rebound tenderness was widespread and he had extreme pain on rectal examination. Could Billy have a real organic problem?

He was admitted to hospital where the surgeon, doing yet another laparotomy, was greeted with an intra abdominal 'sewer' due to a perforated small bowel. Floating on the faeces were two toothpicks and several pieces of silver (Relaxa-tabs in their foil covering).

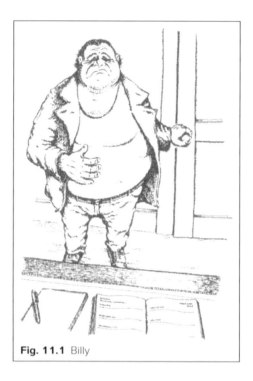

Fig. 11.1 Billy

The postoperative course was stormy and eventually Billy died. Every time I think of this loyal patient and great character, I feel guilty about those fantasies of dispatching him into a tank of piranha fish.

DISCUSSION AND LESSONS LEARNED

- While recognising the obvious lessons it is important that doctors realise they should acknowledge their own feelings and emotions but not permit them to cloud their rational management of patients, especially when they are most vulnerable (that is, tired, stressed or angry).
- Another trap: familiarity can breed contempt.

If you don't put your finger in . . . !

The variety of foreign bodies which have found their way into the rectum is hardly less remarkable than the ingenuity displayed in their removal. A turnip has been delivered PR by the use of obstetric forceps. A stick firmly impacted has been withdrawn by inserting a gimlet into its lower end. A tumbler, mouth downwards, has several times been extracted by filling the interior with a wet plaster of Paris bandage, leaving the end of the bandage extruding, and allowing the plaster to set.

Bailey and Love's Short Practice of Surgery, 1943, p. 1020

WB, aged 74, presented with eight weeks of vague ill health and intermittent abdominal discomfort. He described a feeling of lethargy, malaise, anorexia and nausea, abdominal colic with bloating and unsatisfactory bowel evacuation. On specific questioning about his bowel function he described an unusual pattern of constipation and episodes of diarrhoea with unexpected soiling of his underwear especially when he passed flatus. He also had difficulty passing urine with frequency and a poor stream. He had not lost weight and there was no family history of gastrointestinal malignancy.

His abdomen was moderately distended but there was no specific area of tenderness or organomegaly. On rectal examination there was a mass of hard faeces in a patulous rectum and smearing of faeces around a dilated anus. He had a moderately enlarged, firm regular prostate. A diagnosis of faecal impaction and spurious diarrhoea was made and I prescribed Coloxyl tablets and a Microlax enema.

On review two days later he said that he had better bowel actions but 'something isn't right in my back passage'. On rectal examination most of the faecal mass had gone but I could feel a really hard mass and something really sharp in the mass. It had me puzzled and as I was thinking about taking an abdominal X-ray and a rectal evacuation under general anaesthesia, part of the mass broke and gave way. I was then able to manipulate out the rest of the foreign body and it was the bony carcass of a duck. He then informed me that he was a keen duck shooter and that he and his duck hunting mates would have a good feed of their catch by the river and wash it down with lots of beer. His eating and swallowing habits must have been remarkable as is the human gastrointestinal tract, but it was still hard to explain. I had removed some extraordinary objects that had been introduced into the rectum but this was something new.

DISCUSSION AND LESSONS LEARNED

- Constipation with faecal impaction is common in general practice and sometimes the diagnosis requires lateral thinking as patients, particularly the elderly and infants, can present with poor health and abdominal discomfort. Patients, especially the bed ridden, debilitated and cognitively impaired, may be unaware of the state of their bowel problem. The presence of spurious diarrhoea may be an important clue.
- It is important to do a rectal examination in a patient (especially elderly) presenting with incontinence or urinary retention.
- We should keep in mind the ageless medical aphorism: 'If you don't put your finger in it, you put your foot in it'.

Twin trouble

A 39-year-old patient who presented with a history of six-week amenorrhoea and mild pelvic pain was ordered a pregnancy test that was found to be positive. Pelvic examination revealed an enlarged uterus consistent with dates, but no other masses or tenderness. I had delivered her first baby in 1990 and she had a termination of twins at eight weeks' gestation in 1991.

On the phone a few days later she complained of further pain, and an ultrasound examination was organised. This confirmed a six-week uterine pregnancy with demonstrable cardiac activity. In the left ovary there were two small cystic areas consistent with a *corpus luteum*.

The abdominal pain became more severe and she presented to the surgery where she was seen by one of my colleagues. She had vomited twice, had loose bowels, and was found to be hypotensive. Her blood pressure was 70/50 with a tachycardia of 100 per min. Abdominal examination showed tenderness and guarding and she was transferred to the emergency department of a nearby hospital where she became shocked, developed shoulder tip pain and required oxygen and intravenous resuscitation. The diagnosis seemed to be of an ectopic pregnancy, but investigations had proved negative. Fearing rupture of an abdominal viscus, I consulted a surgeon, who was also puzzled by the diagnosis and performed a laparotomy through a McBurney's incision.

A ruptured ectopic pregnancy was found with 1.8 L of blood in the pelvis. By this time her haemoglobin was 6 g/dL and she required a blood transfusion.

On review with the radiologist the following day, he still felt that there was an intrauterine pregnancy. A repeat ultrasound was performed, confirming a continuing viable intrauterine pregnancy. Subsequent scans showed significant growth. The eventual outcome was a good story.

DISCUSSION AND LESSONS LEARNED

- Always think of ectopic pregnancy until proved otherwise in a woman of childbearing age with abdominal or pelvic pain and early amenorrhoea, irrespective of negative investigations. The 'classic' picture of ectopic pregnancy includes abdominal pain and a history of amenorrhoea and vaginal bleeding; however, early presentation may be atypical. It has been estimated that up to 50 per cent of ectopic pregnancies are misdiagnosed at initial presentation.

- Twin pregnancy should also be kept in mind.
- Be mindful of the value of pelvic ultrasound and quantitative beta HCG (human chorionic gonadotropin) testing.

Inherited 'suntans'

Roger, a 19-year-old student, presented with fever and vague upper quadrant abdominal pain during convalescence from a bout of influenza. His mother rang to say that he was an 'unusual yellowish colour'. I immediately thought he probably had hepatitis or infectious mononucleosis.

When I saw Roger the striking feature was an unusual suntan (for the mid-winter), but he had mildly icteric sclera that was noticeable when he was taken outside to the sunlight. He claimed that the colour of his urine and stools was normal. The only abnormality on his liver function test was an elevated bilirubin of 55 mmol/L (normal less than 17).

Diagnosis and outcome

I realised that Roger probably had the relatively common Gilbert's syndrome, which is inherited as an autosomal dominant trait. Temporary rises of bilirubin occur with intercurrent infections such as influenza, episodes of fasting and strenuous exercise.

I then realised that Derek, his father, had a permanently highly coloured complexion. Tests confirmed that he also had Gilbert's syndrome. Fortunately, it is a benign disorder and so reassurance was the appropriate management.

DISCUSSION AND LESSONS LEARNED

Gilbert's syndrome is a common and benign disorder that can be sitting under our clinical noses, perhaps forever, without a diagnosis. Its recognition is important to avoid unnecessary repeated investigations and perhaps even surgery.

Not an easy game

One of the essential skills of the ever-learning and practising general practitioner is the ability to pick up the signals. These signals will be flashed at any time on any day of any week amid a great variety of often mundane clinical material presented. They may happen frequently or infrequently, in singles or in runs; they have no respect for public holidays, Monday morning brain fog, or the Friday afternoon dreamtime, and they have no respect for the time of day . . . as these authentic case histories show.

An unexpected outcome

'Doctor, could you come to see Albert? He's rolling about and says the pain in his tummy is terrible.' It was just at the end of evening surgery and everything had seemed tidily tied up.

I set off, mentally rehearsing the patient's history as I drove the short distance to his home: committee man, ardent Mason, keen Rotarian—background of cigarette emphysema, two years ago had a RIND (resolving ischaemic neurological defect), known chronic duodenal ulcer and secret whisky imbiber.

When I arrived he was rolling about and looked dreadful. The onset had been sudden, as he was about to go to a Rotary dinner, and he was obviously not suffering a perforation. He was tender throughout and bowel sounds were numerous.

The betting was between bowel obstruction and pancreatitis. A phone call to our usual surgeon resulted in admission, and confident, conservative

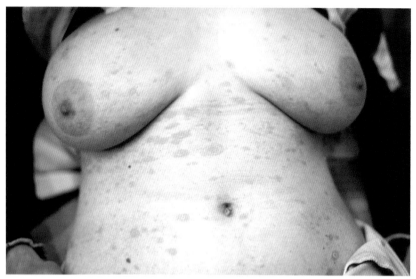

Fig. 2.3 Josie: Pityriasis rosea. *See page 29*

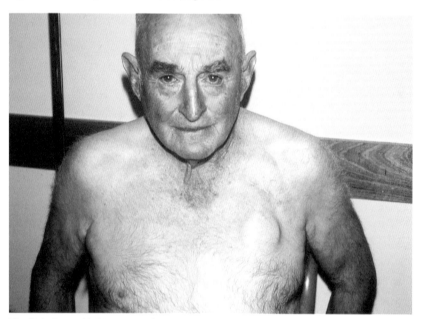

Fig. 3.1 Sam with his pacemaker, which solved his recurrent blackouts and dizzy spells. *See page 36*

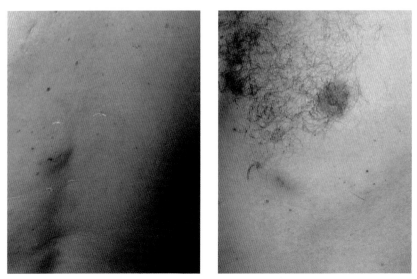

Fig. 3.3 Herpes zoster of T7 dermatone with separate lesions on chest and back. *See page 44*

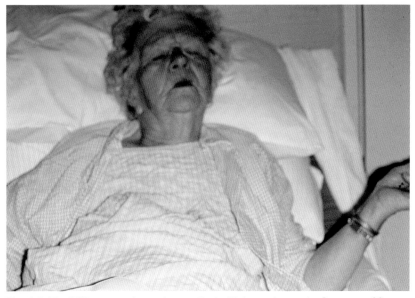

Fig. 4.1 Mrs Williams: semiconscious patient with hypoglycaemia. *See page 62*

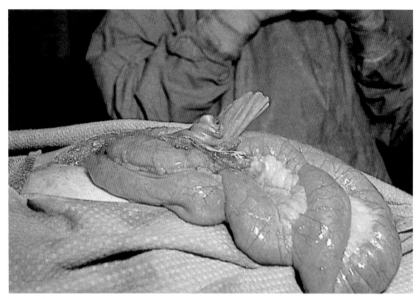

Fig. 6.1 Corrugated drain tubing left behind accidently following a cholecystectomy 21 years previously. *See page 102*

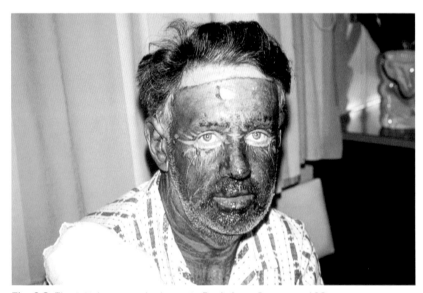

Fig. 6.3 The initial gunpowder burns to Ron's face. *See page 108*

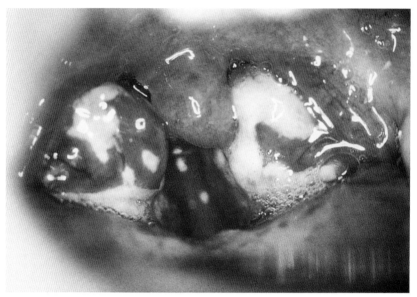

Fig. 7.1 View of throat showing 'tonsillitis' of Epstein–Barr mononucleosis. Photo courtesy of Hugh Newton-John. *See page 117*

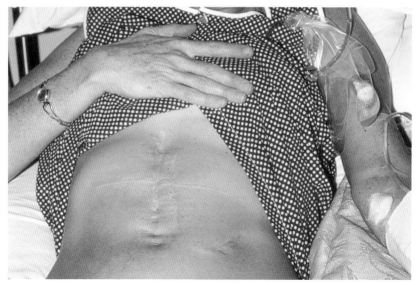

Fig. 7.3 Sheryl in hospital showing multiple scars on abdomen. *See page 124*

4

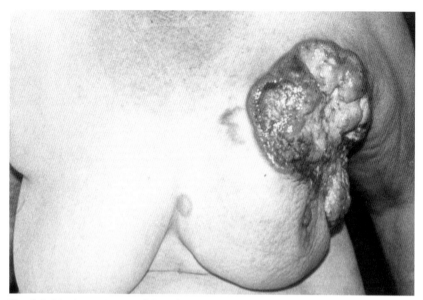

Fig. 9.1 Mrs A: carcinoma of the left breast. *See page 147*

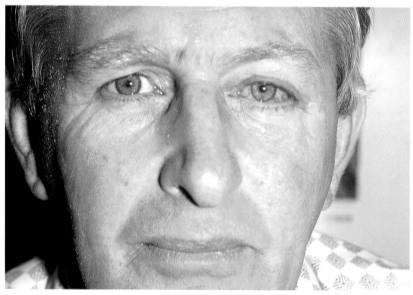

Fig. 11.2 Alan with conjunctoval congestion due to a carotico cavernous fistula. *See page 171*

5

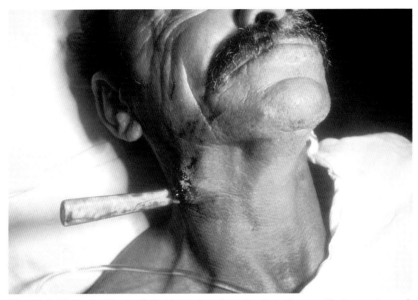

Fig. 14.1 Michael with a knife in his neck, referred pain to the ear. Photo courtesy of Bruce Black. *See page 202*

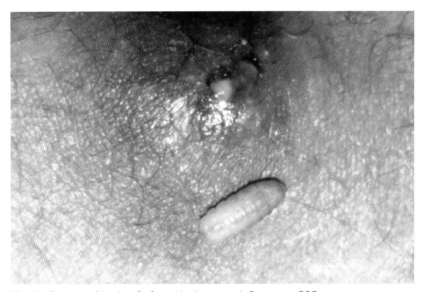

Fig. 14.2 Larva of the bot fly found in the wound. *See page 206*

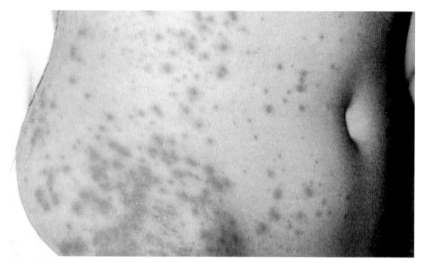

Fig. 14.3 ND with pseudomonas folliculitis. *See page 207*

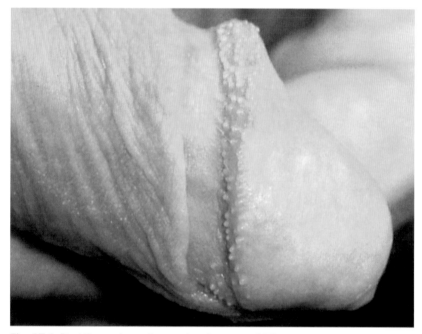

Fig. 15.1 David's pearly penile papules. *See page 217*

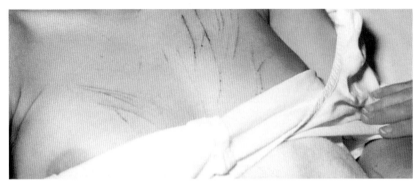

Fig. 20.1 Self-inflicted injuries with a sharp knife. Photo courtesy of Professor David Wells, Victorian Institute of Forensic Medicine. *See page 280*

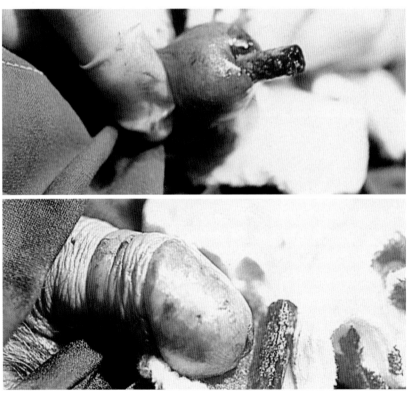

Fig. 20.2 The pencil being extracted from the penis. The pencil was 3cm long and the patient had removed the lead before inserting it. *See page 285*

management of a likely pancreatitis was expected. Then a sudden change of tack was called for. His condition deteriorated and urgent laparotomy revealed a large section of gangrenous small bowel tucked in a corner—an unexpected outcome.

Second time is easy

During that same evening surgery our GP registrar had asked me to look at a man with a unilateral leg swelling and associated peculiar rash. Sure enough, this man in his early 30s had a pale, swollen leg with some bruising. His own doctor a few days earlier had diagnosed a simple injury, yet there had been no trauma and beside the 'bruising' there were a few small purpuric spots—the 'telltale' spots.

Next morning the haematologist phoned to confirm a 'hairy cell' leukaemia.

'We'll start him on interferon—the drug that has been looking for a disease for years. At last it has found one.'

Our GP registrar had gone numb thinking about the implications of the diagnosis. The week before we had seen an 8-month-old boy with 'bruising'. A few days before, he too had been seen by another doctor who, after careful examination, had concluded that it must be simple trauma. Blood examination had revealed a dangerously low platelet count.

Diagnosis always seems easy the second time around.

An additional clue

Mr B had complained of a change in his bowel habit. He had done this before and investigation had been negative. Nonetheless, one must always abide by the rules, and so barium enema was performed and no neoplastic lesion identified; all seemed well.

Later Mr B came to see my partner. He now had pain in his lower abdomen and his social life had been wrecked because he always felt 'ready to go'. Sigmoidoscopy was performed, and a large lesion was identified in the sigmoid colon and resected. Reporting back to base with an additional clue saved his life.

Developing a 'nose'

Wilhelm, an ageing Dutchman, had told me of the spots he could see before his right eye. Vision seemed fair on my examination—'floaters' seemed a reasonable answer.

Luckily, GPs (like Agatha Christie's Hercule Poirot) develop 'the nose', and a hunch that something was not quite right pushed me to phone our favourite ophthalmologist. A small retinal tear was identified and repaired that same night.

DISCUSSION AND LESSONS LEARNED

- During our weekly discussion it was pointed out to our GP registrar that in general practice one must never develop the 'Dr Kildare syndrome'. Problems do not come one at a time, to be solved once a week in episodic fashion. They attack from all angles at the same time; each one has to be resolved and they have to be resolved in parallel. Having dealt with one problem the GP has then to go out and 'face the next ball'.

- General practice may be compared to a complex game. There are problems to be solved and approaches can vary. The answer may be in a spot diagnosis or perhaps logical steps. You may get a second chance, especially when provided with an additional clue. It may be that a hunch or second thoughts set you on the right track, or you may be lucky enough to take advantage of an opponent who has missed the vital clue on first confrontation, and, of course, the answer and solution may be totally unexpected. Complex indeed—general practice is not easy.

An unkindness of cancers

There is a variety of clinical material in day-to-day general practice, both in life and in death. We may also see such variety within particular groups and conditions. One of the most commonly feared is cancer. And to make things even more unpleasant and difficult, the initial presentation may not direct the unwary observer towards the dreaded result. Things may not be what they at first seem.

Those who follow the writings of Ruth Rendell will be aware of the collective word for a group of ravens included in the title of one of her books: *An Unkindness of Ravens*. I think this collective noun is most appropriate to describe the cases I am about to present: 'An unkindness of cancers'.

Don

He had just finished a half-marathon. His training schedule had been a bit hurried and incomplete, and so he was not surprised to feel unusually tired at the finish of a gruelling morning's run. Yet Don was a bit alarmed by the severity of the headache and the fact that his spoken words emerged scrambled. Although not his usual doctor, I did not mind having a look when asked. I had known for years that he was always fit and healthy. Everything seemed normal, and so we jointly agreed to a diagnosis of a badly organised training schedule.

A few weeks later, this formerly healthy young man with two grown-up daughters had an epileptic fit. He was taken to hospital and after investigation found to have a brain tumour that turned out to be highly malignant. It all began as a post-exercise headache.

Fred

In his late 50s, Fred had been a top-class sprinter all his life and continued this pastime into veterans' athletics. Life-long bronchiectasis made his training schedule even more determined. After the World Veterans meeting in Melbourne in 1987, he set off with his wife on a driving tour of Tasmania. He found the driving extremely difficult because of the severe back pain that had developed. On returning home, Fred went to his trusted chiropractor and his physiotherapist. The pain steadily worsened until the nights became sleepless. By the time I saw him his face was grey and lined and his abdomen grossly distended. I phoned our favourite surgeon. Fred was operated on that night and within 24 hours we knew he had a highly malignant, inoperable renal neoplasm, unlikely to be sensitive to radiotherapy or chemotherapy. All within a month.

Clare

Life had not been particularly kind to Clare. Mother of five children, she had been widowed by 40, when her husband, Merv, had a myocardial infarction.

Life indeed was not easy. Then came interest and a sense of purpose in the form of a new job—a marriage celebrant.

On Monday morning, Clare presented with severe diarrhoea. It all seemed straightforward—a food-caused infection. The diarrhoea persisted, the pain was very severe and the culture was negative. I sought the opinion of a gastroenterologist: no inflammatory disease, no bowel neoplasm, carry on as before. Clare became worse; this time she seemed very tender in the left upper quadrant with the definite possibility of a mass. Laparotomy showed widespread ovarian neoplasm. The long, hard road of chemotherapy loomed ahead. All from an attack of severe diarrhoea.

Jenny

Full of zest and exuberantly healthy, Jenny had just returned from interstate to become secretary to one of Queensland's chief executives. Married with no children, significant illness had been unknown in her 39 years.

She presented one Saturday morning with a cough, wheeze and a slight fever. 'They have all got this one down South!' The expected abnormal chest noises were heard and an antibiotic carefully prescribed.

Two weeks later, Jenny returned. This time she looked most unwell; gone was the healthy glow. 'I am no better and get easily puffed when jogging.' The chest sounds had changed. Now one side was completely silent—collapse? Infiltrate? Chest X-ray appearances were sinister, and the subsequent thoracotomy revealed a large inoperable mesothelioma. This was in a healthy, non-smoking, active young woman with no history of asbestos exposure. All were devastated.

Three months later on New Year's Day, Jenny died—in the end, death came rather suddenly. All from an apparently simple respiratory infection. 'From simple beginnings' indeed.

DISCUSSION AND LESSONS LEARNED

- The unusual presentations of these four cases remind us once more that the game we general practitioners have chosen to play is not an easy one. We must be ever listening and watchful.

- Jenny's death came mercifully quickly, but for Don, Fred and Clare, all three diagnosed late in the year, only one thing is certain—neither they nor their families can look forward to a happy immediate future.

An impossible hole in the head

Alan H, a 51-year-old truck driver, fell from the back of his truck onto the road of a Sydney suburb in 1977. After regaining consciousness 10 hours later in a hospital, he complained of a 'banging' sensation in his head behind the left eye.

He was examined by several doctors including two neurologists who, with the benefit of several X-rays, informed him that apart from a massive 'black eye' there was nothing seriously wrong with him.

When he reported to me 10 days later he complained of a persistent 'banging' behind the left eye, loss of balance (intermittent), headache (intermittent) and a floating sensation when lying on his back.

Diagnosis and outcome

Although I had never encountered it I wondered if Alan had developed a carotico cavernous fistula. On inspection he had a large resolving periorbital haematoma and congestion of the conjunctival vessels of the left eye. (Refer to Figure 11.2, centre insert page 5.) With the stethoscope I could hear an unmistakable high-pitched bruit over the eye and at any site on the left half of the face and forehead.

I referred Alan to a neurosurgeon who confirmed the fistula by cerebral angiography, but he said surgical intervention was ill advised and Alan would have to learn to live with his problem.

Alan found this decision incomprehensible in an age of wondrous medical technology but bravely confronted the problem, which he admitted was 'driving him mad'. He was forced to give up his work and hobbies. Aeroplane travel was impossible: 'I felt my head was going to blow off my shoulders'.

I was called out of the cinema dramatically one evening to attend a family crisis: Alan was attempting to 'murder' his wife. Fortunately, it turned out to be only a token gesture but its significance was inescapable. Alan and his family required constant support. I contacted the neurosurgeon who still refused to operate. Alan had to face the daunting prospect of a banging in his head—100 000 times a day—for the rest of his life.

When Alan moved to a town 80 km away the local general practitioner phoned me to say he could not cope with Alan and his problem and was returning him to my care, despite the distance.

I scanned the literature and did a literature search but could not find an answer. Then I saw a glimmer of hope while listening to a brilliant young ophthalmologist speaking at a 'Recent Advances in Medicine' course. I referred Alan to the ophthalmologist who in turn sent him to a neurologist who contacted a radiologist who recently had acquired the equipment that perhaps could seal the fistula.

The radiologist introduced a large guide catheter into the internal carotid artery. A fine catheter conveying a tiny latex rubber balloon at its extremity was then threaded inside the original one and flowguided—through the fistulous site in the internal carotid artery—into the cavernous sinus. The balloon was inflated with a silicone polymer and detached by a third catheter. The first attempt failed to obliterate the fistula but a second balloon sealed the hole. This technical achievement was a first in eastern Australia, the only other being performed in Perth in 1979. Thus, after four long years, Alan was cured of the banging in his head.

DISCUSSION AND LESSONS LEARNED

- We should not necessarily accept a consultant's opinion as final. They are human and capable of mistakes such as 'missing' a carotico cavernous fistula. The conservative neurosurgeon was correct in his refusal to operate but, sadly, unaware of the availability of new technology.
- Total patient care may mean championing your patient's cause as their advocate and constantly searching for a solution to a difficult problem.
- The tools of trade should be used appropriately and more often. The wonderful stethoscope appears to be an instrument used too infrequently.
- Modern medical technology can offer amazing cures for selected patients: it behoves us to keep abreast of advances.

Worm tales

The big one

One day I received a call from a woman in obvious panic because her nine-year-old son had passed a massive white worm that resembled a small snake. They came to the surgery and indeed the specimen was most impressive and scary to the inexperienced. It was a foot-long (30 cm) roundworm (*Ascaris lumbricoides*). They were reassured that it was nothing unique in rural practice and that he would not be devoured internally (as intimated) by such infestations. A single dose of pyrantel reinforced the issue.

The earthy one

News about the great worm travelled fast in the small community and I understood that there were some nervous inspections of toilet bowls. Eventually an elderly woman presented with a specimen in a jar. It was found in her toilet. It was a common earthworm! This was one of three instances in which earthworms were confused with one of the parasitic nematodes.

The symptomatic pinworm saga

A mother consulted me about 7-year-old Steven who was not settling well at night, had poor sleep and affected school performance. Apparently he would fall asleep and after an hour or so would wake complaining of abdominal colic. And yes, he did also complain of an 'itchy bottom'. I asked her to get a torch and inspect his anal area about an hour after he fell asleep. Mother reported back that she observed small 'threadworms' about one inch (2.5 cm) long. I prescribed a dose of pyrantel. About two nights later a home visit was requested and the outcome was amazing. Steven had passed a large piece of orange peel enveloped by a writhing mass of pinworms (*Enterobius vermicularis*). Experience taught me to consider the possibility of pinworm activity as a cause of unsettled children soon after they fell asleep. Any infestation requires scrupulous hygiene in the family and also a veterinarian check of any pets, especially dogs.

Human threadworms

Mary was a federal policeman's wife who had spent 18 months accompanying her husband on his tour of duty in Southeast Asia. Before leaving she had been diagnosed as having polymyalgia rheumatica and was taking corticosteroids to control her pain. Upon returning home she consulted me because she felt so miserable, with a myriad of symptoms which included recurrent abdominal pains with diarrhoea and anorexia. She said that the illness started with a pruritic maculopapular rash on the feet and then she developed a dry cough and wheezing which has persisted on an intermittent basis. On examination she looked unwell, with Cushingoid features and a swollen abdomen without localising signs and no skin lesions. First line investigations were a chest X-ray (negative), a stool micro and culture (negative) and a full blood examination which showed significant eosinophilia. In view of her immuno-compromised state I consulted a tropical diseases expert who was most concerned about a hyperinfection syndrome from *Strongyloides* (human threadworm) or hookworm.

Further investigation confirmed infestation with *Strongyloides stercoralis*. Apparently diagnosis is difficult because eggs and larvae are seldom found on random stool examination. Diagnosis may depend on finding larvae on duodenal biopsy or a specific ELISA (Enzyme-Linked Immunosorbent Assay) test. Treatment is with ivermectin or albendazole.

DISCUSSION AND LESSONS LEARNED

- *Strongyloides* (human threadworm) is a prevalent parasite, especially in tropical and sub-tropical countries.
- It can live and reproduce in the body for many years.
- High-risk people include migrants and refugees from tropical developing countries, returned soldiers, and workers or residents in northern Indigenous communities.
- The problem is aggravated by corticosteroid therapy and may present as a severe infection such as septicaemia.
- The infestation may be asymptomatic but it can cause abdominal pain and swelling, and diarrhoea, skin and respiratory symptoms.

Sheepish business

Wally McGregor, a Bendigo GP, describes the case of LK, a 22-year-old farmer and elite footballer who presented with a 12-month history of right shoulder tip pain aggravated by the bouncing motion of a tractor and playing sport. LK had seen several doctors, including specialists, without a diagnosis. Wally ordered imaging, which was normal, and on review the patient complained of pain in the right hypochondrium where tender hepatomegaly was found. Because his family owned a sheep farm, a Casoni test was ordered (no specific imaging was available at the time) and it was positive for *Echinococcus* (hydatid disease). LK then had instillation of formalin (a scolecoccidal agent) into the hepatic cyst, followed by partial hepatectomy and is still well a generation later. Sporadic cases of *Echinococcosis* still occur and I have seen it recently in a person who spent many months in Thailand and Mongolia.

Chapter 12

Sacked and rejected

'Sacked'

Mrs Roberts

Last Tuesday morning Mrs Roberts was admitted to one of the local nursing homes. This slightly surprising news was conveyed by the nurse manager, asking if I could continue her care. Mrs Roberts was one of my regular home visits, a lifelong battler, loving mother and grandmother.

Her hypertension had eventually been too much for the cerebral arteries and she suffered a severe stroke with permanent hemiplegia. Her retired husband had taken on the role of permanent nurse, but unfortunately he succumbed to a heart attack; we were left with one devoted daughter to take on the burden of carer. With much weeping, the caring daughter, who just could not cope, had sacked herself as permanent carer.

Mrs Thomas

Sacking was very much in my mind as I thought over a year of dismissals. In the field of government, the Queensland electorate had just sacked the long-reigning National Party. Doctors can also be sacked by their patients.

It occurred to me while driving that I had not seen Mrs Thomas for some time. A regular patient, Mrs Thomas had suffered from multiple complaints, including osteoporotic fractures and a very high ESR, the cause of which several colleagues and I had failed to track down. She was one of my 'specials' with numerous problems that I never quite managed to cure or relieve fully. She did, in fact, become one of my 'first-division heartsink' patients. However, we had become used to one another, which is one of the developments in the care of the 'heartsink', and regular consultation and counselling seemed to be meeting with good reception and some success, or so I thought. With the thought, 'Where are you, Mrs Thomas?' in my head, one of my spies (yes, GPs do develop their very own networks) informed me that Mr and Mrs Thomas had been seen quietly slipping off in the direction of another practice in the district. What had I done wrong?

Myrtle and Alice

That same week, I had been taken aback early on the Monday morning by one of my long-standing famous doubles: ancient women from the parish. 'Your services are terminated, Doctor,' said Myrtle with her eyes staring straight ahead. 'Thank you for your help in the past.' End of conversation. This couple I had considered my very own forever. Was I losing my touch?

Mrs Jackson

Only a month previously I had received a little note from another practice asking if I would, please, send some details about Mrs Jackson. 'Mrs Jackson?' thought I. 'I only saw her last week. I have looked after her for 11 years. We had a good relationship.' Obviously not good enough.

Nothing daunted, I picked up the phone. 'Mrs Jackson, we have known one another a long time. Before I say goodbye could you tell me if you were totally dissatisfied with my care?'

'No, Doctor, but I felt you didn't want to follow up investigation about that last problem I had and I thought you should have. My husband and I discussed it.' (He had given me up a long time ago.) 'He suggested it was time for a change.'

When you have been in an area a long time, events like these happen regularly in general practice. I do not make a habit of seeking reasons for patients 'changing channels' but I must admit to being a bit miffed on this occasion. Nevertheless, it is the patient's privilege and after all we live in a free country. I often wish I had the courage to advise patients to go elsewhere—but that's another story.

DISCUSSION AND LESSONS LEARNED

- Why do patients change their doctors? The reasons are legion—dissatisfaction over a particular illness or death; difficulty in getting an appointment; on holiday at a time when the patient needs you; new face in the practice or in the district; falling out with reception staff; part of the grief reaction; widow rejection; embarrassment at personal or marital problems; mutual breakdowns of previously good vibes; or perhaps they simply become tired of your face or your personality.
- Whatever the reasons for this change of direction, it does no harm to pause just a little and think. And yet we must not become paranoid. However, if feeling particularly paranoid and pipped, remember these words wisely written by Shakespeare in *Hamlet*:

  > *This above all: to thine own self be true,*
  > *And it must follow, as the night the day,*
  > *Thou canst not then be false to any man.*

The widow's rejection

Like Isaiah's God, the general practitioner must become 'a man [or woman] of sorrows and acquainted with grief'. The general practitioner is privileged because the nature of family practice brings direct involvement with a relatively constant group of people over a long time. This gives exposure to a broad gamut of human emotions: boredom and excitement, worry and relief, joy and sadness. There is opportunity to experience vicariously the whole of life from birth to death.

A demanding aspect of patient management for the family doctor is terminal care in a home environment, in particular when a man is cared for by his wife. In my experience this can lead to another phenomenon seen only in general practice which I call 'widow rejection': a sudden and obvious dismissal—a coldness in attitude toward the attendant doctor—by the new widow. The once-friendly and (self-confessed) dependent woman apparently terminates the relationship; the expected and inevitable death of the husband creates a post-mortem distance, which might never be bridged.

Is this phenomenon real or imaginary? Is it oversensitivity by the doctor in what is an emotional situation? I think it is real.

Case 1

Mr C, a retired builder, lived with his wife in an attractive cottage with a large garden area; their only daughter was in another part of the country. I attended him through progressive cardiac decompensation: hypertension; ischaemic heart disease; severe angina; attacks of paroxysmal nocturnal dyspnoea; total cardiac failure; and then a slow orthopnoeic death. His care demanded much attention day and night for months. The couple had insisted on terminal management at home without nursing help and it became distressing for both of them in the end.

Mrs C seemed cold toward me thereafter.

Case 2

Mr R and his wife lived in a well-furbished villa unit. They were most fond of each other, although she was the dominant partner and could be demanding. Their one child, a son, had been estranged for some time.

I had been their family doctor for years when Mr R developed cerebrovascular atherosclerosis with gradually increasing dementia, although at first he was merely absent-minded and forgetful. My visits became more frequent.

Death was sudden. Mrs R remarried not long afterwards and no longer sought my counsel.

Case 3

Mr and Mrs D were comfortably placed and lived in a pleasant home complete with swimming pool. They had no children and late in married life adopted twins. Mr D was a heavy smoker and, as seemed almost inevitable, developed lung cancer. I had looked after them always and this couple, too, insisted on terminal care at home. Mrs D did all the nursing; they were very close and he wanted no one else involved. The deterioration was protracted and painful, but my frequent visits and the use of opioids ensured the final stages were not too distressing for any of the family.

However, Mrs D saw me infrequently afterwards.

Case 4

Mr and Mrs S had escaped across the Balkan frontier during a snowstorm one night in 1945. Their daughter lived at a distance and a strong bond endured between them through their hard-working life into (finally comfortable) retirement. Mr S had long-term vascular problems; hypertension had led to vertebrobasilar insufficiency and then peripheral vascular disease. His only hope of avoiding leg amputation was arterial bypass surgery. Despite the risks of anaesthesia, the vascular surgeon and I pushed for the operation. He came through it successfully but did not survive a postoperative cardiac arrest.

Mrs S refused to accept his death and the once warm relationship with her GP was terminated.

How can we explain such rejection?

On review of these cases, a pattern emerges. Two people are close to each other for a mixture of reasons: they are childless or have only one child at a distance; or share a background of emotional and physical hardship. These circumstances have led to a particularly interdependent relationship, usually with a dominant female partner allowing a 'third party' to care for her failing spouse. A *ménage à trois* of sorts is formed.

DISCUSSION AND LESSONS LEARNED

The examples illustrate the evolution of an unhealthy situation in medicine. An attempt should have been made to involve others—a partner in the practice, social worker, district nurse—so that the burden could be spread more widely. The stricken couple might resist such a suggestion, but I see no other way to prevent a tolerable situation becoming one of soul searching, paranoia, hurt and resentment.

Misunderstood medical comments

Mrs B, a prim and unmarried lady, was a regular and loyal patient whom I noticed had ceased attending the practice. One day when I was consulting her sister I enquired after her health and was informed: 'Doctor it's very embarrassing but I should tell you that she took offence with your diagnosis'. Sacked! Without further clarification I realised that I had said 'Your problem is intermittent claudication'. I suspect the following explanation fell on paralysed deaf ears. Once again proves the value of a patient education hand-out.

101 obstetric ways to be sacked

Obstetric care is arguably the most wonderful and satisfying aspect of general practice. The immense satisfaction of sharing the joy of the birth of a precious, wanted child is one of the privileges and highlights of our great profession. The experience can cement a special bond between the family and their doctor. However, sometimes the events do not match anticipations and this has led to the author being 'sacked' by new mothers, sometimes with just cause, other times without.

Case 1

Liz was a 30-year-old primigravida who had been having difficulty conceiving. Some special treatment solved the problem and the baby was awaited with great excitement. However, Liz was one week overdue when her blood pressure started to rise. I decided to induce labour, admitted her to hospital and ruptured the membranes. About five minutes later she started to get strong contractions, coinciding with my departure to theatre to reduce a Colles' fracture and then suture a large laceration. About an hour after rupturing the membranes I was called to the labour ward to be confronted with an amazing sight. The midwife was anxiously holding back the visible head of the baby. Quite delighted, I took over and made a neat episiotomy out of the beginning of a posterior tear. The baby was then expelled like a rocket into my arms. I apologised about the lack of analgesia but commended her on her labour.

I was subsequently sacked! She informed the nursing staff that she was unimpressed by my attention (or lack of it) during the first stage, and by my behaving like a goalkeeper rather than a skilled *accoucheur.*

Case 2

Rachel, a 26-year-old multigravida and schoolteacher, came into labour with her second child after coming into my care only two weeks previously. When I performed a pelvic examination during the second stage I felt the soft presenting part of a breech (or so I thought). I then informed Rachel that the baby was coming bottom first but everything would go smoothly. To our surprise and distress an anencephalic baby delivered. I hastened the baby out of the room before it cried and then had the difficult task of explaining the problem to the stunned parents.

I was quietly dismissed and the family travelled a long distance to another town for medical attention.

Case 3

Barbara, aged 34, gravida 3, presented in advanced labour. Pelvic examination felt different in that the membranes were intact but the head well down. Next thing a bulging membrane came in to view and baby was delivered covered in its membrane. The last time I had encountered a caul delivery was as an intern in an obstetric hospital. Barbara looked stunned at the strange sight, but I explained that everything was fine and then passed some mythical quip that 'your son will never drown'.

I was sacked from further obstetric care.

Case 4

I had just completed the smooth second stage of 25-year-old Christine's first baby when the attending nurse pointed out that she had lost only a few drops of blood. The delivery area was amazingly dry and so I decided to do without ergometrine for the first and only time in my career. She was still 'dry' at the end of the third stage. About one hour later I returned to assess the patient and noted that she was pale and sweaty. 'Her observations are not good—she's not well.' On palpation of the abdomen the uterus was found to be greatly distended. It was full of blood. The emergency required the usual dramatic routine of ergometrine, inserting an IV line, organising a blood transfusion and emptying the uterus.

That was the last time I omitted to give ergometrine and the last time I attended Christine. Sacked! Perhaps deservedly so.

DISCUSSION AND LESSONS LEARNED

- Obstetric care is an emotional and sensitive phase in a woman's life. Sometimes the patient can be most forgiving of less than optimal care; other times they feel cheated when normal expectations are not met. I have learned to give full explanations of any deviations from normal and not pass 'smart' remarks.
- I have always given ergometrine on the delivery of the baby's shoulder ever since that awesome postpartum haemorrhage where bleeding occurred into the uterus and not *per vaginum*.
- Despite these upsetting incidents obstetrics remains a special part of medicine. Most confinements are smooth and incident free, yet the occasional one can cause much anxiety and stress. Being prepared, with appropriate skills and equipment (especially blood) available, and watchful will cover virtually all contingencies.

From gossip to online

Patients are increasingly discussing their medical care online. From time to time patients will post critical comments about the care they have received and even sack their doctor online.

Dr D was 'Googling' his name when he came across the following review about him:

> *The worst GP I have ever seen. Dr D was rude, arrogant*
> *and disinterested. It was like I was wasting his time. Never*
> *see Dr D if you are ill—or well.*

Dr D was understandably distressed. He didn't know who had posted the comments online and wanted to know what he could do to have them removed.

DISCUSSION AND LESSONS LEARNED

- It is important to obtain support and advice in this situation—the lack of control and public shaming of online criticism can be extremely distressing. There is often very little that can be done to remove, or even respond to, negative online posts. Options include:
    - do nothing
    - if you can identify the person who has posted the comment, consider contacting them directly to discuss their concerns and see if they will remove their comments
    - utilise the website policy for removal of posts
    - post an online response but be careful not to breach confidentiality; do not post in anger and ensure the reply is appropriate. It is a good idea to discuss this with a colleague or your medical defence organisation
    - consider legal remedies, such as defamation proceedings.
- It is also worth reflecting on the comments to identify if there is any constructive criticism to assist you and your practice to improve patient care.

Musculoskeletal twists and turns

Chapter 13

Myalgia beyond tolerance

Susan, a 39-year-old fashion designer, presented because of very severe pain in her lower back and legs. The problem followed a febrile illness of sudden onset following a recent business trip to Singapore and Thailand. She had attributed the pain to a recurrence of an old problem of sciatica and was concerned that she may have been infected with swine flu. Two days before our appointment, she had visited an emergency department for pain relief and was prescribed oxycodone because Panadeine Forte was ineffective. She said that now the pains in her legs were unbearable and not responding well to opioids. Further detailed history revealed that she had associated fever, malaise, nausea, headache and generalised muscular aching. She also admitted to feeling very depressed—even suicidal. On physical examination there were no specific musculoskeletal or neurological signs (despite the severe pain), just a temperature of 38.2 °C.

As tears streamed from her eyes describing the unbearable pain in her thighs and lower back, the term 'breakbone fever' went through my mind. Blood tests confirmed dengue fever which is caused by a flavivirus transmitted by the *Aedes* mosquito.

DISCUSSION AND LESSONS LEARNED

- Dengue fever is widespread in the south-east Pacific and endemic in Queensland. A returned traveller with myalgia and fever < 39 °C is more likely to have dengue than malaria.

- A similar tropical infectious disease is chikungunya, which should be considered.
- We should use caution with opioids in diseases causing temporary myalgia.
- Depression with suicide has been reported in troops with dengue fever fighting in the tropics.

The painful knee: search north

Tom B, a 51-year-old timber worker, presented for yet another opinion about his painful right knee. The knee had been getting increasingly painful for about two years and now the pain was so severe he could not complete a day's work. Apart from being considerably overweight, Tom looked fit and well.

I could not detect any abnormality around the medial aspect of the knee where Tom claimed to experience 'terrible pain'. An accompanying X-ray of his knee was normal. He said that he had visited three doctors, including a specialist who said that his knee probably had early osteoarthritis. NSAIDs had helped but not in the past few weeks. I wondered about nerve entrapment or referred pain from his spine (L3) but could not find any abnormality.

Diagnosis and outcome

I referred Tom to an orthopaedic specialist as I had known Tom from my days in the bush and believed that his pain was genuine. The specialist rang me and said, 'You've fallen for the old trap. He has severe osteoarthritis of the hip and will need a hip replacement. You should have known better.' Tom was a very happy person when surgery of the hip relieved the pain in his knee!

DISCUSSION AND LESSONS LEARNED
- Hip joint pathology can cause referred pain in and around the knee without pain in the hip. We must always check the hip joint in such patients, especially in adolescents presenting with knee pain and a limp for a slipped upper femoral epiphysis (Figure 13.1).

- A good working rule is to examine the lumbosacral spine, hip and knee for patients with pain in the upper leg from pelvis to knee.
- The hip joint is innervated by L3.

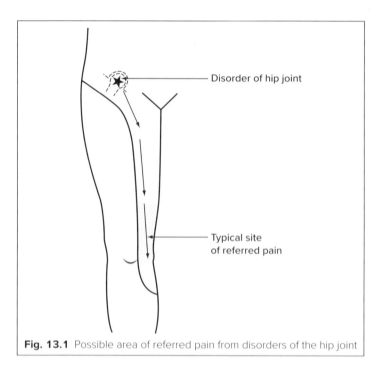

Disorder of hip joint

Typical site
of referred pain

Fig. 13.1 Possible area of referred pain from disorders of the hip joint

The thumb that pulled out a lemon

With its extensive range of movement the thumb is unlike any other digit on the hand and injuries to it also tend to be unique. To choose the correct treatment (often a surgical one) requires special understanding. Of particular concern are injuries to the two major joints—the carpometacarpal and the metacarpophalangeal.

Filip the cheesemaker

Filip, a 46-year-old Lebanese cheesemaker, was upset because his painful left thumb was not responding to treatment. Six weeks previously, while holding the handle of a cheese-scraper between his thumb and second finger, a heavy blow resulted in a sudden hyperabduction and extension force to the thumb. He immediately reported to the factory medical officer.

Diagnostic possibilities

Filip could have ruptured the ulnar collateral ligament of the metacarpophalangeal joint with or without avulsing a bony fragment—the 'gamekeeper's (or skier's) thumb'. It could be diagnosed clinically with instability on radial flexion but X-rays with stress views would confirm the diagnosis. It is a relatively urgent surgical problem because early treatment gives optimum results. He could have a fracture dislocation (Bennett's fracture) of the base of the first metacarpal. This is diagnosed radiologically and reduction is necessary before immobilisation.

The first six weeks

The industrial medical officer arranged a routine X-ray of the thumb and the report offered '. . . suggestive of early osteoarthritic degeneration of the carpometacarpal joint'. Filip was given analgesics for a 'strained thumb'. Follow-up therapy included topical and oral anti-inflammatory agents and physiotherapy.

Our first consultation

Filip came to me complaining of a deep, burning ache in his thumb; examination revealed swelling, tenderness and heat at its base. His ESR and serum uric acid level were normal, and so I referred him to an orthopaedic surgeon who diagnosed ligamentous injuries of both major joints of the thumb. He decided surgical exploration was inappropriate and prescribed plaster immobilisation for four weeks.

The 'compensation merry-go-round'

That strategy failed and Filip began a series of visits to consultants, most of whom were insurance company doctors. Eventually, an enthusiastic plastic surgeon convinced him an operation would solve his problem. Six months after the accident Filip's trapezium was removed and replaced by a Silastic implant.

It was not the answer. The problem deteriorated and he was dismissed as a 'compensation neurotic'.

Review

Filip came to see me again, looking most depressed. He had lost his job; his thumb ached; a deep, burning pain, which often enveloped the whole arm, had developed in his wrist. The fingers were stiff and the overlying skin was discoloured, becoming cyanosed when dependent. He noticed increased sweating of the hand and wrist.

Filip had reflex sympathetic vasodystrophy (now known as complex regional pain syndrome). An X-ray showed spotty demineralisation of the bones. He was referred to a pain clinic, but a stellate ganglion block and several other treatments were unsuccessful.

More than two years later, Filip was handicapped by a disabled left hand. His troubled hand returned to normal about three years post-injury.

DISCUSSION AND LESSONS LEARNED

- It is critical that the doctor of primary contact recognises serious ligamentous disruption of joints and arranges early surgical referral.
- In retrospect, the syndrome of reflex sympathetic vasodystrophy was apparent at our first consultation. It is commonly misdiagnosed, and it can follow only relatively minor trauma.
- The inappropriate label of 'compensation neurosis' is to be deplored, especially as an alibi for professional frustration or ignorance.

A 'lost' grand final

Twenty-seven-year-old Robbie, a timber contractor who worked in the bushlands of Victoria and Tasmania, was a fine athlete, outstanding Australian Rules footballer and champion axeman.

He was the key ruckman in the football team of the country town where I practised medicine. Football was the town's 'religion': cultural, social and drinking life focused around the sport. Unfortunately, Robbie was plagued by recurrent soreness in the anterior compartment of his right leg, especially when the playing surfaces were dry and hard. Localised tenderness at the musculotendinous junction of the tibialis anterior muscle in the lower third of the leg was diagnosed as tendonitis. I advised rest and then packing the area with ice after playing sport.

The town was struck in the spring by an infectious disease known as 'finals fever'. (No one was spared—not even the doctor.) Robbie presented two days before the grand final with acute tenderness over the tibialis anterior which exhibited crepitus on movement.

The team's fate depended on Robbie's participation and I was uncomfortably aware of 2900 supporters breathing down my clinical neck. Reluctantly, I infiltrated the tender area with one per cent lignocaine (15 mL) immediately before the game and at the half-time interval. Robbie played an inspired game and the local team became premiers (the celebrations still rage many years later).

When I next treated Robbie, for a different problem, he related an amazing medical tale.

His work had taken him interstate the year after his football triumph and the lure of the sport led him to join the town's team. Predictably he 'starred' and they qualified for the grand final.

Robbie's right tibialis anterior ached terribly. He consulted the local doctor who had arrived recently in Australia from another continent and could not understand this strange game, football. Although bemused by the problem, he agreed to administer a painkilling injection before the final match.

Robbie reported to the surgery an hour before the game and, to his surprise, the injection was given into his arm. He was not impressed. 'I don't want that injection again, Doctor,' he told me. 'I felt quite strange, as though I was a spectator rather than a participant; I played like a zombie. It was a disaster.'

The substance? Pethidine.

DISCUSSION AND LESSONS LEARNED

- Do not encourage injections of local anaesthetic in sports men and women to 'prop them up'.
- Do not given them parenteral injections, especially opioids.
- Provide patients with their history when they move elsewhere, even if only temporarily.
- If athletes have a persistent problem with the anterior compartment of the leg, refer them to a consultant or hospital: surgical intervention could be appropriate.

By heck, watch the neck!

The cervical spine is the origin of many confusing clinical problems such as headache, migraine-like headache, arm pain, facial pain, periauricular pain, anterior chest pain and even visual dysfunction and dizziness. If the cervical spine is overlooked as a source of pain (such as in the head, shoulder, arm, upper chest—anterior and posterior—and around the ear or face) the cause of the symptoms will remain masked and mismanagement will follow. The following case histories illustrate such problems.

Case 1

Nellie P, aged 39, was a charge nurse who presented with a seven-year history of unilateral headaches. They were migraine-like, associated with neck ache, and they appeared to follow a motor vehicle accident. After four years under the care of a neurologist she spent three years under a psychiatrist having psychotherapy for functional headache. My partner determined that it was referred from the left side of C2–C3 and administered one cervical manipulation after performing a Hallpike manoeuvre as a safety precaution. The headaches disappeared completely never to return (to date).

Case 2

Tania B, aged 36, was a regular attender with multiple complaints especially 'migraine' headaches, which were unusual in that the headaches could last three days or so and occurred at least weekly. We had just completed a D and C for excessive uterine bleeding and were shifting her from the operating table onto the trolley when her head flopped to one side with a huge, resounding 'crack'. We were most concerned about this wrench in her neck but relieved when she awoke with no ill effects. When she presented in about three months she said, 'Well, my bleeding hasn't improved much but I can recommend a D and C for migraines. I haven't had one since'.

Case 3

A 59-year-old woman was referred by a colleague for cervical manipulations because she had a six-month history of pain radiating down the arm to the fingers diagnosed as a C6–C7 disc lesion. I agreed to see her although I was not prepared to manipulate a neck with nerve root pain. On examination the pain and anaesthesia affected three nerve roots C6, C7 and C8. Remembering the golden rule one disc, one nerve root, I conducted a more searching examination and found several large, shotty nodes deep in the axilla. Biopsy revealed lymphoma.

Case 4

A minister's 62-year-old wife was referred because of a four-month history of pain and paraesthesia in the right hand, which was worse at night. She also had severe neck pain and headache. The first X-ray showed degenerative changes. She was diagnosed as having carpal tunnel syndrome but decompression of the carpal tunnel was unhelpful. Cervical manipulation aggravated the problem and also brought on tingling in the left hand. Examination confirmed weakness of both C6 and also C7 nerve roots. A CT scan revealed destruction of the C7 vertebrae with an obvious malignancy, probably secondary to carcinoma of the kidney removed five years previously.

Case 5

Margaret B, aged 43, an American tourist, presented with an episode of severe vertigo, which she said had bothered her on and off for the past five years since a motor accident. After spells of being well, the bouts could be precipitated by actions such as collecting overhead luggage from a plane. She had associated headaches but no nausea or vomiting. She marvelled at the wonderful tests performed at the University of Birmingham (USA): scans, MRI (Magnetic Resonance Imaging), angiograms and so on, but they all showed zero. She produced Persantin tablets and Stemetil tablets for the treatment of alleged spasm of her cerebral arteries and inner ear inflammation respectively. On examination she had an extremely tender C2–C3 level of her neck and it appeared that the problem could be benign positional vertigo associated with cervical dysfunction. Since vertebrobasilar inefficiency tests were negative I performed mobilisation and a gentle rotational manipulation with resounding effects. Seven months later I received this letter from Goodwater, Alabama:

> *I have sung your praises to all who will listen. I have not been bothered with inner ear ever since you gave me that adjustment. I arrived at the conclusion that it isn't inner ear in all cases.*

DISCUSSION AND LESSONS LEARNED

- Dysfunction of the cervical spine can cause many unusual symptoms such as headache and vertigo, a fact that is often not recognised. Despite teaching to the contrary from some consultants, the cervical spine is a common cause of headache, especially dysfunction of the facet joints at the C1–C2 and C2–C3 levels.
- Expert mobilisation or manipulation of the cervical spine can be a dramatically effective technique, but it should be used with care and never used in the presence of organic disease and vertebrobasilar insufficiency. It should, therefore, be given only by skilled therapists. Two groups at special risk from quadriplegia are those with rheumatoid arthritis of the neck and those with Down syndrome because of the instability of the odontoid process.
- If pain or anaesthesia in the arm involves more than one nerve root look for other causes (one disc = one nerve root).

Gout in little, old, religious ladies

Maude S was a very prim and proper 75-year-old lady with a past history of congestive cardiac failure who presented with very painful fingers. On examination she had nodular deformities including Heberden's nodes of the fingers. X-rays confirmed osteoarthritis and I prescribed NSAIDs. She returned with exacerbation of her cardiac failure, which I attributed to the fluid-retaining property of the NSAIDs; I increased her frusemide and ceased the NSAIDs. She then consulted me with worsening of her arthritis. The distal interphalangeal joints were red and swollen, and she complained of terrible pain in her right great toe.

The penny dropped! It was gout. Foolishly, I then inquired about her alcohol-drinking habits, apparently in an accusatory manner. This went down like a 'lead balloon' to an entrenched member of the temperance society. I was slow to appreciate that the frusemide was the cause of the hyperuricaemia.

DISCUSSION AND LESSONS LEARNED

- Do not jump to conclusions, and treat sweet little old ladies as you find them.
- Gouty arthritis can flare up in osteoarthritic joints, especially in the hands and feet—the so-called 'nodular gout'.
- Frusemide, in addition to the thiazide diuretics, can precipitate gouty arthritis known as 'diuretic gout'.

Beware the fall from a height

Milos, a 63-year-old lawyer, presented to the clinic because of extreme difficulty walking following an accident on a ladder at home. The ladder slipped from the house gutter and he was forced to let go and land on his feet (particularly the heels). By the time he was seen, weight bearing was not possible because of pain in the right heel which looked wider and flatter when viewed from behind. There was tense swelling of the heel, marked local tenderness and a D-shaped bruise under the foot. I organised X-ray examination which included anteroposterior, lateral (most important) and mortice views of the ankle as well as a calcaneal axial view.

When he was being moved to the X-ray room he complained of pain in the back at the waist level. Further radiology of the pelvis and spine were ordered. The radiographs revealed an intra-articular fracture of the calcaneum involving the subtalar joint, fracture of the pelvis and a compression fracture of T12.

DISCUSSION AND LESSONS LEARNED

- Falls from a height onto the feet can lead to a complex of injuries to the skeletal system. These include fractures of the calcaneum, talus, tibia and fibula, pelvis and vertebrae especially at the thoraco-lumbar junction. For this reason in the patient presenting with a fracture of a calcaneum investigate the opposite calcaneum, ankle, pelvis and spine. CT scans are appropriate to provide clearer imaging of the degree of calcaneal fracture and any subtalar and calcaneocuboidal joint involvement.
- Other associated injuries to consider are central dislocation of the hip, fractures of the radius and ulnar bones and even concussion.
- This traumatic injury complex is commonly encountered in slaters, window cleaners and construction workers. Those undertaking home maintenance involving climbing ladders are also at risk. People over 65 years are advised not to work on ladders.

Sniffing out the 'anatomical snuffbox'

Multiple cases of a painful wrist

While I was serving on secondment to the Australian Army caring for conscripted national servicemen during the Vietnam War, a young man fell off an army tank and sustained a fractured scaphoid which led eventually to his discharge from the unpopular program. Subsequently the medical centre was flooded with men presenting with the complaint of a painful wrist with a pointing sign to the 'anatomical snuffbox'. The complaints were bogus but it kept us 'on our toes'.

William was a fit 22-year-old apprentice who sustained multiple minor injuries following a fall off his motorbike. He returned to the hospital which treated his injuries; he complained of pain in his hand, centred on the lateral aspect of his wrist. The pain had seemed to settle in the weeks after hospital in-patient care but returned with activity. His hand was examined in the emergency department where it was diagnosed as a wrist sprain and treated with a supportive bandage. The discomfort persisted and when he visited our clinic we observed the following signs on examination:

- tenderness in the anatomical snuffbox
- loss of grip strength
- swelling in and around the snuffbox
- pain on axial compression of the thumb towards the radius.

The clinical diagnosis of a fracture of the carpal scaphoid was verified by X-ray.

DISCUSSION AND LESSONS LEARNED

- William's case eventually became a medico-legal issue which is reasonably commonplace with scaphoid fractures and a cause for concern and care.
- A scaphoid fracture is caused typically by a fall on the outstretched hand with the wrist bent backwards (dorsiflexed). The pain may settle after the injury so presentation may be later. One has to be careful not to treat it as a simple sprain.
- If a fracture is suspected clinically but the plain X-ray is normal a fracture cannot be ruled out so an MRI scan or isotope bone scan is helpful after 24 hours post-injury. If scans are not available, immobilise the wrist in a scaphoid plaster for 10 days, remove it and then re-X-ray. An oblique scaphoid view, in addition to an anterior–posterior and lateral view, is required.
- For an undisplaced stable fracture immobilise for eight weeks in a below-elbow plaster cast. Displaced fractures require reduction (either open or closed) and, if unstable, internal fixation. All fractures require a later X-ray to check for non-union.

Special senses

The eyes have it: six short case histories

The following case histories of interesting eye problems have presented to the authors.

Case 1: Ian M, aged 30, motor mechanic

Ian's wife rang me at 2 am with a suggestion of panic in her voice. Ian was extremely distressed, with agonising pain and 'burning' of both eyes: he felt he was going blind. Mrs M could think of no reason for his eyes to be affected this way. He had been perfectly fit and well when he went to bed. A distressed Ian groped his way through the surgery door. On examination, his eyes were very red but there was no discharge.

Case 2: Jim W, aged 56, fisherman

Jim presented because of deterioration of vision in his right eye during the previous six weeks. The sight in his left eye was good. The right eye felt hard and the pupil was dilated. Visual acuity was 6/60R and 6/9L (Snellen chart). Intra-ocular tension 28 mm Hg (Schiøtz tonometer)—right eye. Ophthalmoscopy revealed a vitreous haemorrhage and an apparent retinal detachment. The clinical picture was very confusing and so I arranged an urgent appointment for him with an ophthalmologist.

Case 3: Bruce D, aged 42, dentist

Bruce's left eye had been painful for two days. There were no other symptoms and his vision was satisfactory. He had three small superficial ulcers on the lid margins and mild conjunctival hyperaemia but no other abnormal findings. He returned the next day saying his eye was worse and his vision was blurred now, despite using the prescribed chloramphenicol ointment.

Case 4: Craig F, aged 10, rascal

Craig presented with an intolerance of sunlight, especially in his right eye, and his parents had noted the pupil was larger than the left. He was otherwise well and there was no history of trauma. The right eye revealed a fixed dilated pupil; the other was normal.

Case 5: Wendy M, aged 10 weeks, baby

Following grandmother's prompting, Wendy was brought along by her mother because her left eye was 'different': the pupil was enlarged and was a different, unusual colour. Mrs M had noted also that Wendy had not smiled yet; her sister, by that age, had. On examination the findings were confirmed with the left pupil showing a yellow light reflex. She was referred to an ophthalmologist.

Case 6: Yasmin H, aged 5 months, shy

Yasmin's mother was concerned that her daughter was 'afraid of the light' and her eyes were red and watery. Eye examination was difficult and the red eye reflex could not be observed. Referral to an ophthalmologist was made at which time the corneas were noted to be cloudy and enlarged.

Diagnoses

1. Ian M had 'flash burns' caused by watching a builder doing some arc welding that day. The pain was due to an oedematous corneal epithelium and blepharospasm caused by exposure of the unprotected eye to the intense ultraviolet light from the oxyacetylene torch.

Remember this possibility for any patient who rings during the night because of burning and 'blindness' in the eyes. Dramatic relief can be obtained by instilling local anaesthetic. It is advisable to check also for corneal damage and visual acuity. Never send the drops home with the patient. Review next day.

2. Jim W had an intra-ocular malignant melanoma. The intra-ocular bleeding had caused his blurred vision but possibly the retinal detachment had prompted his attendance. The eye was removed and a prosthesis inserted. At a check-up three months later massive hepatomegaly was found: he died shortly after.

   We all learned in medical school the old saying 'beware of the man with a glass eye and a big liver!'

3. Bruce D had a herpes simplex infection with a dendritic corneal ulcer. It responded to idoxuridine ointment and debridement of the ulcer by a consultant.

   Whenever we see painful ulcers we should think of herpes simplex. Fortunately, steroid drops were not used.

4. Craig F had instilled some of his mother's atropine eye drops, prescribed some time ago for acute iritis. At first he denied doing so but persistent questioning by his mother resulted in a confession, much to this doctor's relief.

5. Wendy M had a retinoblastoma in the left eye with an associated retinal detachment. She presented with the classically described 'cat's eye' reflex. In 30 per cent of patients the condition is bilateral and in Wendy a smaller tumour was identified in the right eye, causing impaired vision and hence delayed social development.

   Treatment included enucleation of the left eye and radiotherapy to the right, as well as parental counselling because of the significant genetic influence of the condition. An autosomal dominant gene is involved, and so Wendy's older sister required screening.

6. Yasmin H had bilateral infantile glaucoma. Fortunately prompt surgical treatment resulted in a good visual outcome.

DISCUSSION AND LESSONS LEARNED

- We have to be forever vigilant with problems of the eye, especially with rare tumours affecting the eye, retinal detachment, herpes simplex and herpes zoster.
- Any unusual deterioration in vision demands urgent referral.

An awful earful

George, a general practitioner of 60 in excellent health, developed preauricular pain in the left ear. With a self-made diagnosis of 'a dental problem', he went to the best dentist he knew. The dentist proclaimed the pain was arising from the left temporomandibular joint due to malocclusion of the teeth, which a special dental plate would rapidly solve.

Despite the plastic contraption in his mouth, George found the pain in and around the ear was becoming intense and there was now a feeling of fullness. He asked his partner to have a look at it and was amazed to learn the external canal was swollen and tender. Visualisation of the tympanic membrane with an auriscope was not possible and regional lymphadenopathy was noted. Their revised diagnosis was a furuncle of the external canal requiring penicillin.

During the ensuing 48 hours the pain became excruciating—'like someone dragging barbed wire around in my ear'. George began to suffer with tinnitus, deafness in that ear, fever and lethargy.

Then, two days later, the 'toxic' George developed a staggering gait and collapsed to the floor. The general practitioner who was called identified ataxia, nystagmus, unilateral sensorineural deafness and a temperature of 39 °C.

Diagnosis

On admission to hospital George asked to see a priest. His feeling of impending doom was reinforced by the dramatic development of a facial nerve palsy (lower motor neurone type) and the soft whispers among the gathering relatives: 'Poor George. It was a stroke'.

A more detailed but painful examination of the ear was achieved by forcing the auriscope through the swollen canal. Vesicles typical of herpes were observed on the posterior wall of the external auditory meatus. George had Ramsay Hunt syndrome, a herpes zoster affliction of the seventh and eighth cranial nerves, easier to diagnose early if the vesicles involve the pinna. A consultant considered George also had involvement of the brain stem. Fortunately, an acyclovir infusion produced a rapid recovery.

DISCUSSION AND LESSONS LEARNED

- A proper examination clinched the diagnosis. It is important to look at all relevant anatomical structures—even if it causes considerable discomfort to the patient—particularly if the ear is involved.
- Self-diagnosis in doctors is not recommended.
- Consultation with a specialist who is restricted to one health discipline can result in 'tunnel vision', leading to delays in diagnosis and treatment.
- The Ramsay Hunt syndrome is extremely painful.

Unusual causes of ear pain

A series of brief case histories

1. Jack M, aged 63, underwent a surgical repair of a para-oesophageal hiatus hernia via laparoscopy. The surgery was complex, with difficulty performing fundal plication. He experienced severe post-operative pain in his right ear and it continued for two years, with exacerbations upon eating, especially spicy food. The cause was injury to the vagus nerve.
2. Mohammed A, aged 17, presented with persistent earache but no abnormality of the ear could be found on examination. A dental cause was suspected and radiography confirmed the presence of an unerupted wisdom (third molar) tooth. Extraction relieved the ear pain once healing of the wound occurred.
3. Mavis N, aged 67, complained of increasing ear pain in addition to gastro-oesophageal reflux related to a hiatus hernia. Diagnosis was referred pain from the vagus nerve.

4. Charlotte R, aged 57, presented with brief spasms of severe lancinating pain in the left ear and back of the throat with radiation to the adjacent ear canal. The cause was glossopharyngeal neuralgia, which is neuralgia of the ninth cranial nerve and associated branches of the vagus nerve.

5. Michael, aged 43, presented with a knife injury to his neck. (Refer to Figure 14.1, centre insert page 6.) The resultant laryngeal trauma caused troublesome left otalgia. The cause was referred pain from the vagus nerve.

DISCUSSION AND LESSONS LEARNED

- The common cause of a painful ear is otitis media (in particular), otitis externa or eustachian tube dysfunction. Direct examination of the ear with the otoscope will usually find the cause. However, a red tympanic membrane is not always caused by otitis media. The blood vessels of the drum head may be engorged from crying, sneezing or nose blowing.

- If an adult presents with ear pain but normal auroscopy, examine possible referral sites namely the temporomandibular joint, mouth, throat, teeth and cervical spine. Significant causes include parotitis (e.g. mumps), temporal arteritis, and carcinoma of tongue, palate, tonsils and larynx. An orthopantomogram may help in these cases.

- Referral from cranial and cervical nerves can cause ear pain. These include the maxillary branch of the trigeminal (fifth cranial), facial (seventh cranial), glossopharyngeal (ninth cranial), vagus (tenth cranial), hypoglossal (eleventh cranial) and cervical nerves 1, 2 and 3. The vagus nerve has a potential rich source of referral with auricular branches in the jugular fossa, pharyngeal and laryngeal branches in the neck, left recurrent laryngeal and oesophageal branches in the thorax and gastric branches in the abdomen.

- Herpes zoster of the sensory branch of the facial nerve causes severe pain in the skin of the ear canal—the Ramsay Hunt syndrome.

Pruritic skin rash beyond tolerance

Natasha, a 20-year-old university student, presented in June 2010 with a five-day history of extremely itchy skin lumps on her lower abdomen and right thigh. She had no other symptoms and claimed to be in good general health. On examination there were several red maculopapular wheals arranged in groups of four or five in an orderly line corresponding to superficial blood vessels. There was local swelling and scratch marks.

The patient had just returned from an eight-week backpacking trek from Cairns to Melbourne. She said that one of her travelling companions had also complained of a red itchy rash on her neck and upper arms.

The diagnosis is bedbug (*Cimex lectularius*) bites. This is a classical presentation with the red lesions clustered in a line along superficial blood vessels as the little arthropods suck blood from their sleeping victim. Clinically the bites are usually seen in children and teenagers. The lesions are commonly found on the neck, shoulders, upper arms, torso and legs.

Natasha was not happy about the diagnosis of bedbug bites and infestation, stating that it represented an unhygienic condition. Furthermore she thought that bedbugs were a feature of the dark ages and had become extinct.

A bedbug infestation can be diagnosed by the identification of rust-coloured specimens collected from the infected residence or sleeping items such as mattresses and sleeping bags.

The treatment, which is symptomatic, is as follows:

- Clean the bites with water and perhaps antiseptic.
- Apply a simple anti-itch agent such as calamine lotion, which may be sufficient.
- Most cases are treated with corticosteroid ointment.
- An ice pack will help to relieve swelling.

DISCUSSION AND LESSONS LEARNED

Bedbugs have certainly made a comeback and are currently in pandemic proportions with a particularly high prevalence in the USA. I explained to

Natasha that the infestation is usually acquired by sleeping in places where the bedbugs have been carried by other humans. This is usually in dwellings with a high occupancy turnover such as hotels, motels, hostels, shelters and backpacker accommodation. The bugs hide by day and become active at night. They are attracted to heat and carbon dioxide, not dirt.

Pruritus sine materia ('itch without physical substance')

Taking a history to help pass your oral exam

This case history highlights the importance of a thorough general history involving five simple general symptoms to arrive at the diagnosis. This particular case (or similar) has been presented at several examinations where the pass rate was only about 50 per cent because these routine questions were not asked.

Antoinette

Antoinette, a quiet 16-year-old schoolgirl, presented to me in my first week in rural practice (January 1970) with a two-year history of intermittent pruritus of the trunk. The itch was getting worse over time and causing her to lose sleep. She had consulted her GP a few times, another neighbouring GP and a locum. She was referred to a dermatologist who had seen her two or three times and conducted skin tests. The working diagnosis was that of an allergic dermatitis, probably to duck eggs or mouldy hay on the farm. She had been prescribed an antihistamine (Avil), amylobarbitone and prednisolone in varying combinations. I felt so sorry for this poor girl who had suffered for so long and I was determined to get to the bottom of her illness. I mentally recalled the list of causes of generalised pruritus that I learned in medical school and considered one diagnostic hypothesis from the list before taking a history.

The response to the quintet of general questions was as follows.

Q1. Do you feel tired, lethargic or weak?

A. Yes, the tiredness and lack of energy is gradually getting worse but I get very little sleep with the itch.

Q2. Do you have any fevers or night sweats?

A. Yes—especially at night when I feel hot and sweaty but it comes and goes.

Q3. Have you lost or gained weight?

A. I have lost some weight (mother chipped in to say that she was concerned about her weight and appetite).

Q4. Have you noticed any unusual lumps?

A. I think that I have a lump in the side of the neck.

Q5. Have you noticed any unusual pain anywhere?

A. No, but I think pain might be better than the itch.

The history did reinforce my working hypothesis that Antoinette did have Hodgkin lymphoma. Examination confirmed the presence of two rubbery lymph nodes in the posterior triangle of the neck. A biopsy of one of the lymph nodes confirmed the diagnosis. Our sweet girl was soon in the care of an oncologist and the course of radiotherapy and chemotherapy initiated. He did give a relatively poor prognosis and I recall visiting the family one evening to present a positive approach with the understanding that Hodgkin lymphoma was one malignancy that was potentially curable. Antoinette eventually enjoyed a long remission.

I was looking through the paper's death notices and noted that she had died in December 2010 at the age of 57, almost 41 years after diagnosis.

DISCUSSION AND LESSONS LEARNED

- Persistent pruritus demands thorough evaluation.
- A patient should not have to endure such a delayed diagnosis and a merry-go-round of reviews.
- Using the quintet of general questions as outlined is a very helpful diagnostic strategy, especially for a vague or complex problem.
- In my experience our consultants set very high standards but, occasionally as in this instance, we encounter 'duds'. Our responsibility to our patients is

to refer to first-class clinicians and if a choice of a few excellent consultants is available refer to the one with the lower fees. Patients tend to judge us by our choice for a higher opinion.

- This patient did have in time the classic Pel–Ebstein fever pattern of Hodgkin lymphoma with a few days of high fever regularly alternating with days to weeks of normal or sub-normal temperature.

An unwanted Caribbean souvenir

Simon, a 30-year-old 'sports tragic', returned from a fascinating World Cup cricket tour in the Caribbean with a puzzling skin lesion. It was a painless tumour about the size and appearance of an egg on the dorsum of his lower forearm. He consulted the travel clinic where the doctor, bemused by the lesion, diagnosed an infection and prescribed antibiotics. Following no response he was referred to a surgeon who excised the tumour and found a 2.5 cm-long object. Simon then presented the object to me for identification and it was obviously the larva (maggot) of the bot fly, which is active in Central America where Simon had taken an additional tour. (Refer to Figure 14.2, centre insert page 6.)

I have seen cases of cutaneous myiasis due to fly-blown open wounds but this furuncle (boil-like) myiasis was quite different (Kitching, 1997).

DISCUSSION AND LESSONS LEARNED

- Be aware of cutaneous myiasis (furuncular or wound types) in travellers returning from tropical Africa or South/Central America.
- First aid involves the application of Vaseline to the closed lesion as this may cause the larva to move to the surface and be easier to extract. Another option is to inject local anaesthetic in and around the lesion, make a small incision and extract the larva with forceps.

Summer and *Pseudomonas*

Miss ND was an 18-year-old student with no relevant allergic or medical history. She presented in mid-summer with a history of general 'unwellness' for two days, an itchy erythematous papulo pustular rash, mainly on the trunk, and fever of 38.2 °C. (Refer to Figure 14.3, centre insert page 7.) A presumptive diagnosis of acute folliculitis was made and after taking swabs for micro and culture I started her on erythromycin 250 mg orally, four times a day, and Pinetarsol baths. On review the next day she was afebrile and normotensive, but the rash had not improved; she was sweaty and complained of nausea and generalised aches and pains.

It was decided to admit her to Fairfield Infectious Diseases Hospital, Melbourne, for further investigation and treatment. Cultures had grown no pathogens so far. On admission her condition deteriorated and she became very ill and toxic. A clinical diagnosis of *Pseudomonas folliculitis* was made and she was commenced on intravenous piperacillin and tobramycin for 36 hours and then oral ciprofloxacin. She made an excellent recovery, although the scars took some months to settle. Culture confirmed *Pseudomonas aeruginosa.*

DISCUSSION AND LESSONS LEARNED

- The cause of this severe folliculitis? Two days before presenting, Miss ND had spent many hours in a hot spa bath with eight friends, five of whom became unwell and developed mild rashes. All settled with no treatment.
- *Pseudomonas folliculitis* is a not uncommon phenomenon associated with the use of hot water spas and tubs—fortunately most cases are not as severe as Miss ND's.

Oh for a suntan!

Thirty-three years ago, Pam, then a 25-year-old surveyor, was newly married. She had always enjoyed holidays at her parents' beach house, spending her time sailing and swimming. Her tan was the envy of her friends.

On return from Surfers Paradise in July, she was particularly brown, having spent most of the holiday on the beach. Since her marriage, Pam had been complaining of tiredness and appeared particularly thin. This was attributed to the strain of her professional responsibilities, the demands of an active social life and the stress of starting a new home.

A respiratory infection resulted in profound weakness and lassitude; she collapsed while on the toilet and was unable to shake off the symptoms— despite adequate rest and medical care. She remained in bed for several weeks. She was seen by a consultant physician and admitted to hospital for investigation. All tests proved negative and she returned home only to be prostrated with what appeared to be a simple cystitis.

Her general practitioner observed that although olive-skinned, Pam was inordinately tanned and he suggested adrenal hypoplasia may have been the cause. Pam was seen by an endocrinologist who made a clinical diagnosis of Addison's disease and confirmed this with cortisol assaying. Pam has remained well on replacement therapy for the past 33 years.

DISCUSSION AND LESSONS LEARNED

- In retrospect, everyone realised Pam was browner than her friends. She had always been tanned, however, the gradual deepening of her skin colour went unobserved even by her family, which included several physicians.
- Sir William Osier was a firm believer in the powers of observation and it behoves us as physicians to stand back and look at our patients. We may often learn more than is revealed through sophisticated testing.

The mountain maid

One Sunday afternoon I received an urgent call from the Ski Rescue Service on the nearby mountain resort stating that a 17-year-old girl had 'collapsed'. Her problems were headache, tightness in the chest, dizziness, and difficulty with speech, walking and breathing. The first aid attendant thought she had 'mountain sickness' (hypothermia). Her condition was deteriorating despite treatment, yet she was still conscious.

There was a blizzard on the mountain where the task of transporting her 56 km to my clinic began. She was placed on a special stretcher and towed by a snowmobile to the chairlift. The stretcher was hitched to the lift and, with difficulty, the patient was carefully and slowly lowered to the chairlift base where a special Forests Commission vehicle transferred her to a waiting ambulance. With great drama, police escort and entourage, she arrived in my surgery about five hours after the distress call.

Examination revealed an agitated, prostrate girl who could not offer a coherent history. Her vital signs were temperature 36.5 °C, pulse 124 and regular, respiratory rate 26/min and BP 120/75. There were no neurological abnormalities but she indicated that she had paraesthesiae of the extremities and around the mouth.

Diagnosis and outcome

The provisional diagnosis was acute anxiety and 'hysteria' with hyperventilation. We gave her a lot of positive reassurance and encouraged her to breathe into a paper bag. After 10 minutes she sat upright, looking very normal, and enthusiastically accepted an offer of a cup of tea.

The stunned countenances of her anxious entourage were a sight to behold. One of these embarrassed and anxious characters was the young stud who was responsible for provoking this startling chain of events by making unwelcome sexual advances within the snowbound confines of their chalet.

DISCUSSION AND LESSONS LEARNED

- The hyperventilation syndrome, which is a relatively common problem, can have many subtle manifestations and may not present as a carpopedal spasm. It is important that all personnel in first aid situations receive appropriate training in its recognition and management.
- The installation of a phone line to the first aid centre at the resort now provides direct communication, and better, more economical first aid management. Ideally, medical personnel should be manning busy resort areas.
- The other pitfall was that our thinking had been misdirected to the most likely situational problems: altitude sickness, hypothermia or exposure. Tunnel-vision diagnosis is a common trap.

Mountains and molehills

Background

J is a dynamic and colourful 25-year-old sportsman who has won many accolades in football and athletics. This delightful character was starting to worry me during several uncharacteristic appearances over a period of about eight weeks for relatively trivial complaints, mainly of a musculoskeletal nature.

His problems included headache, neck pain, back pain and groin pain, all of a relatively minor nature with no significant findings on clinical examination. When I confronted him about his general health he admitted to feeling lethargic and uninterested in his beloved sport, claiming that his training program was virtually at a halt. 'I feel stale, Doctor—just can't be bothered.'

I advised J that this flat spot was commonplace in super athletes and that a break in routine, including a 'holiday' to a 'different' training resort would be beneficial. Shortly after this consultation a letter was hand-delivered to my mailbox.

Dear Doctor,

I hope I can take a couple of your precious minutes to discuss a subject that's been a major worry for me for a long time. It is a very awkward and most embarrassing letter to write.

I want to ask you if anything can be done in relation to the size of one's penis. You're probably thinking this is the wish of many a young man; however, I do believe I have a very special case.

All I want to know is can anything be done at all, no matter how drastic the measure need be? It has got to such a stage that it is wrecking my whole life. Many times when I let it get the better of me, my self-concept, my thoughts on the future, etc. are almost zero—completely negative.

It is a constant worry and I know it restricts my total personality. I know it does not directly affect my 'sexual performance', but I wonder now at 25 whether I will ever be able to accept a wife. I know many would say it is a purely psychological thing.

Doctor, I need to know if there is any chance of doing anything to rectify what I believe is an underdeveloped penis, perhaps due to a lack of male hormones during puberty—I don't know.

I know the next step is examination and that will be embarrassing but I thought if I could give you a little time to assess the situation it would be better.

Believe me, it has taken a lot of courage to write this and to confide in you.

The problem

The problem was now obvious, and so I rang J and told him that I had encountered this situation several times in the past. He should not feel too embarrassed about it and should come along one evening so that we could clarify the problem.

J seemed quite at ease during the consultation. The examination did reveal a normal-sized penis albeit at the lower end of the normal range. On direct questioning he did experience normal heterosexual impulses, and did have erections of 11–12 cm. When I asked him why he thought that he was so 'small', he said it was based mainly on comparisons with the other guys in the showers at the change rooms.

A knowing, sheepish grin transformed J's face when I casually said: 'Now you've fallen in love, haven't you? You've probably met your match and you're thinking about getting married and you have some anxiety about your manliness, your sexual performance and your ability to father children'.

'That would be close to the mark, Doctor, but is it possible to carry out a hormone test to make sure?'

A serum testosterone was ordered because I could see that counselling would not reassure him completely. A normal result made him feel relieved and reassured. He gradually regained his confidence and his normal zest for life.

Now, years later, he is happily married with three children and claims that his sporting activities are as enjoyable as ever.

DISCUSSION AND LESSONS LEARNED

- Anxieties about penile size and sexual performance, including the ability to induce conception, are common characteristics of young men, especially when they meet the 'right woman' in their life.
- As general practitioners we should bear this in mind with premarital counselling. One strategy would be to subtly raise the issue by using the third person in an offhanded matter-of-fact manner. For example: '. . . we

find that guys in your situation often worry about their manliness and their ability to be good husbands and lovers'. This approach may trigger open discussion should such an anxiety be significant. Of course, most men are able to dismiss this fleeting apprehension, but for the occasional patient such extreme anxiety manifests itself in frequent and apparently trivial attendance at the surgery.

A novel way to treat pruritus vulvae

Jeanie E, aged 29, presented with recurrent vaginal thrush with an interesting associated effect—insomnia! Upon initial presentation she had the typical cottage-cheese-looking vaginitis and I prescribed nystatin cream.

I repeated this treatment when she re-presented two months later. She then started treating her pruritus vulvae with the cream. After another two months she came in with her husband, both looking worn out and glum. 'Doctor, you'll have to do something about the thrush—I've had it', exclaimed the bleary-eyed husband. 'Jeanie finds that the only relief for her itchy vagina is intercourse. She tapped me on the shoulder three times during last night. I'm not that good.'

'Well, I can't scratch it and sex soothes it at least for a little while,' explained Jeanie.

Diagnosis and outcome

The gauntlet had been thrown down to me to stop the self-perpetuating itch-intercourse-itch cycle. I examined the vagina and could not find any evidence of significant vaginitis. 'I always seem to be itchy now and I've done all you told me: no deodorants, no tampons, no jeans, no pantyhose, no antibiotics.'

I went through my check-list and decided to get her to pass a specimen. Glucose +++. A random blood glucose was 17 mmol/L. The old diabetes had tricked me again.

DISCUSSION AND LESSONS LEARNED

- For recurrent vaginitis, pruritus vulvae or any other skin infection I always think diabetes mellitus. Sometimes, sadly, the 'diabetic thoughts' are sluggish or absent.
- It is amazing the many ways in which diabetes can present without the classic textbook symptoms of polyuria and polydipsia. However, the symptoms may be present when one takes a more searching history.

Marital surprises

The devoted married couple

Mrs CP, a 42-year-old with type 2 diabetes, presented with a several days' history of migratory polyarthritis. Examination revealed a fever, tachycardia, a few non-tender, subcutaneous nodules and a tender, swollen right knee, on which she was unable to bear weight. Initial investigations showed an ESR of 84 mm/hour and raised C-reactive protein. A working diagnosis of rheumatic fever was made and she was admitted for bed rest and treatment with aspirin and penicillin.

We had all noticed the devotion of her elderly husband who sat by her bed almost all day, every day, chatting and doing crossword puzzles. We had also noticed that she had a young male visitor 'waiting in the wings' who would appear only after her husband had gone.

After a week the subcutaneous nodules had disappeared, but the right knee remained painful and swollen and she was still unable to walk. Thus it was decided to aspirate this knee. Imagine our surprise when four days later the laboratory phoned to say that gonococci had been cultured from the joint aspirate. Contact tracing revealed that her husband had not been sexually active for years and she was having a relationship with the young man.

Suspicions alerted

Mrs AT, a 34-year-old, presented 12 days after Mrs CP with a two-day history of fever and pain and swelling of the wrists and metacarpophalangeal joints so severe that she was unable to feed or dress herself. There was no history of illness. On examination, a systolic murmur was detected. I remembered that she had had gonorrhoea six months ago, so in addition to the usual investigations for polyarthritis I took an endocervical swab. While waiting for the results she was admitted and treated with indomethacin, which had little effect on her symptoms. Luckily, the visiting orthopaedic surgeon, who visits every three months, arrived two days later and aspirated frank pus from both her wrists. She was commenced on intravenous antibiotics, but after three days of treatment was able to feed and dress herself and left hospital. Gonococci were isolated from the endocervical swab and joint aspirate.

DISCUSSION AND LESSONS LEARNED

- Relationships between married couples are not always what they seem. Mrs CP and her husband seemed to be a devoted middle-aged couple and this image probably delayed the diagnosis of her gonococcal arthritis.
- Not all illnesses that fit the Jones criteria for the diagnosis of rheumatic fever are rheumatic fever. Both these patients had polyarthritis, fever, raised ESR and C-reactive protein, and Mrs AT also had a raised anti-streptolysin O titre; however, the culture of gonococci from their joint aspirates proved the diagnosis of gonococcal arthritis.

Fretting for mature love

Mrs S was the formidable 81-year-old widowed matriarch of a large family in a rural township. Her dutiful daughter would bring her in for a check-up because she would 'throw wobblies'. Her 'wobbly' was described as a 'turn' or 'space-out' in which she would collapse, become aphasic and sometimes throw her arms around. I could not find any abnormality on examination or investigation. One day I received an urgent call to attend to mother because she was found lying unconscious on the laundry floor. I had to travel 14 km and when I arrived 20 minutes later I could see that there was no sign of trauma and her breathing was normal. Then the prone patient said, with eyes closed, 'Why has it taken you so long?' I realised that it was a conversion reaction (hysteria). Physical examination was normal.

When the family left the room she quietly said (still lying prone with eyes closed), 'What I need is a good man and a good bang'. Her rather naïve young doctor was dumbfounded.

DISCUSSION AND LESSONS LEARNED

- Age does not limit the need for sexual intimacy.
- The loss of a loved partner has more ramifications than we care to consider in our counselling and understanding of grieving.
- We do need to be careful in labelling a patient as hysterical. In conversion disorder or fugue states the cause may be unconscious and the patient is not feigning. The patients often seem far less distressed by the symptoms than would be expected—this is known as *la belle indifference*.

Traumatic sex

I was attending to the immediate post-delivery stage of a complicated obstetric case when the nurse said that a woman had appeared at our small hospital at 1 am with vaginal bleeding. I said to settle her down and I would eventually see her (wondering where I would get norethisterone at that hour!). After about three minutes the nurse returned looking agitated: 'you should come quickly'. I did and found a small 39-year-old single woman who was having profuse vaginal bleeding and her circulation was compromised. She told me that she had been working at a nearby fish and chip shop and after work had intercourse with the boss and the bleeding started soon after. I could see that the bleeding was profuse and coming from the vaginal vault so a large pack was put in the vagina to arrest the bleeding and an intravenous line inserted. Once the poor embarrassed patient was stabilised we arranged for my partner to come and administer a general anaesthetic. Repair of the wound was difficult as there was a 7 cm laceration in the vaginal vault and oozing of blood was profuse. A blood transfusion was required.

DISCUSSION AND LESSONS LEARNED

- Apart from the unseen value of preventive measures we don't actually experience the reward of saving life, but being able to save people by successfully managing acute bleeding is one such rewarding occasion.
- Trauma, both physical and psychological, can be the unfortunate consequence of the simple act of vaginal intercourse and this should be kept in mind.
- The advantage of the availability of a medical team (in this case husband and wife) for emergency work becomes obvious.
- I often recall the interesting quote from cousin Jim, an ex-Inspector of police: 'You know, John, sex will drag you further than gun powder will blow you!'

Pearly penile papules

David, a 22-year-old postgraduate student, presented with what he described as 'a sensitive issue'. It was our first consultation but I knew him as a rather reclusive earnest young man around the district. He came from a very religious family and was a devout Christian. David was embarrassed as he described lumps on his penis that he thought may have been a sexually acquired problem, 'perhaps from toilet seats', although he said that he was a virgin. Inspection revealed the somewhat common problem of benign pearly papules on the corona of his penis. (Refer to Figure 15.1, centre insert page 7.) Upon diplomatic questioning he did admit that he wondered if they were caused by masturbation. However, he was most relieved by the assurance that all was well and he appreciated the opportunity to chat about important facts of life for the first time.

DISCUSSION AND LESSONS LEARNED

- This experience reinforced the importance of appropriate sex education in our young people, preferably by caring parents.

- We need to educate our patients on an opportunistic basis about normal human anatomy, physiology and behaviour, and alleviate any identified feelings of guilt.

A case of mistaken identity

Some medico-legal cases are stranger than fiction, and without any lessons to be learned. This was one of them.

The GP anaesthetist rang me for advice after receiving a bizarre and troubling call on his mobile phone. The female caller had said: 'You had sex with me last night and you didn't pay'.

The GP was aghast and said he had absolutely no idea what the caller was talking about. He asked her how she had got his mobile phone number. The woman replied that he had given her his business card last night after sex in a brothel. The quick-witted GP asked where she was calling from. She said she was in Brisbane. The GP said he did not live or work in Brisbane and he certainly had never had sex with the woman. After some discussion about his physical appearance—'Are you tall and well-built with black curly hair?' 'No, I am short, pudgy and balding.'—the caller was satisfied that it was, indeed, a case of mistaken identity.

It was the routine practice of the GP anaesthetist to give patients his business card post-operatively in case they had any questions or problems. The business card included his mobile phone number and the GP assumed that one of his patients had inappropriately used his card.

Feverish problems

Pyrexia in the cowshed

Nancy, a 58-year-old farmer, presented with a 12-month history
of exertional dyspnoea and angina. When she subsequently
presented with episodes of dizziness, a classic triad came to mind.
Dizziness/syncope + angina + exertional dyspnoea → aortic stenosis
(of course this constellation of symptoms can occur with anaemia). On
auscultation there was the harsh crescendo–decrescendo systolic ejection
murmur of aortic stenosis that would remind me of a steam train chuffing
uphill or distant barking of a dog (strange associations from student days!).

I was concerned and sent her to a visiting physician for an opinion
about further investigation with a view to surgical repair. He thought that the
condition was not sufficiently severe to warrant further investigation, stating,
'we'll still play it by ear'.

About three months later I received a call to attend to an emergency in
the family's cowshed. While milking, Nancy developed chest pain and then
collapsed and was unconscious for a few minutes. As she lay in the fresh
cow manure and mud of the milking shed she looked sick and humiliated and
was hot to touch (her temperature was 38.7 °C). There was no paramedical
service at that time so I performed an ECG with my portable unit. There was
no evidence of an acute coronary ischaemic episode although I could not
exclude it.

I was very concerned and rang the admitting officer of our usual referral
metropolitan hospital to inform him that I would be pleased if he could admit

my patient with the probability diagnosis of subacute bacterial endocarditis. 'What makes you think that, Doctor?' came the response in cynical overtones, as though a remote rural doctor was incapable of such a diagnosis. However, he agreed to admit Nancy, who was transported by a regional ambulance. She was admitted with pyrexia of unknown origin (PUO). After two or three days of procrastination about the diagnosis and management Nancy suffered an embolic stroke resulting in left hemiparesis. It was due to a mycotic embolus from a 'vegetating' aortic valve. All hell and penicillin broke loose! The organism was *Streptococcus viridans*. After seven months she was discharged back to my care with a prosthetic valve, hemiplegia and cardiac failure.

DISCUSSION AND LESSONS LEARNED
- The plight of the busy stressed GP with a seriously ill patient and also the admitting officer with limited available hospital beds is highlighted.
- It could be argued that an experienced general practitioner has a greater diagnostic acumen than less experienced hospital interns and resident medical officers and their skills should be given due recognition.
- The problem of procrastination with serious and potentially life-threatening infections is reinforced yet again. It is sometimes most appropriate for doctors to act as advocates for their patients if they consider that the medical system is not acting with due urgency.
- This case also reinforces the valuable discipline of learning aide-memoires such as diagnostic triads or tetrads which come readily to mind during pressured circumstances, e.g.
  PUO + cardiac murmur ± embolism → endocarditis.
- We should keep in mind that sudden death is a feature of aortic stenosis.

'Yellow face' syndrome

Rosie B, aged 38, was one of those 'heartsink' patients with seemingly perpetual melancholia. She would present with a shopping list of complaints year in, year out, and she had been subjected to several operations of questionable necessity. The underlying cause of her malaise was a poor relationship with her husband whom she described as demanding and a 'sex maniac'. She had an aversion to a sexual relationship with him but would not leave him because she wanted the security of a 'roof over her head' and hung in for the children's sake.

The home visit

One day I was asked to perform the ubiquitous call to her because she was 'feeling extremely ill and had no energy to go anywhere'. I was led into her darkened room. 'I can't stand the light, Doc.' I found her in a similar state to when I am called to treat her migraines. She complained of a moderate headache and of being tired, listless, nauseated, tender in the abdomen and feverish. The history was not typical of migraine but similar to the flu that she had two years previously. Despite the familiarity of the scene I carefully checked her out—no neck stiffness, no specific abdominal signs but a temperature of 37.5 °C. I explained that it was probably an intercurrent viral illness and that she should call me in two to three days if she was not any better.

Second opinion

The usual call eventuated with a comment that she felt worse and would like a second opinion. I agreed and asked my partner to see her. She contacted me later in the day saying that Rosie was jaundiced and probably had hepatitis A.

DISCUSSION AND LESSONS LEARNED

- It pays to keep an open mind when assessing the frequent attender or morbid hypochondriacal patient and look for evidence of organic disease compatible with the symptoms.
- It is a mistake to examine patients in poor light and perhaps artificial light. Yellow skin and conjunctivae can be easily overlooked. The story is often told about troops nursed below the ship's deck whose jaundice went

undiagnosed until they appeared on deck for convalescence. Another tale is told about a famous house physician at St Barts, London, who would quiz his students on where to look for jaundice. He would not accept 'the whites of the eyes' and when the answers from the student group came to an impasse he would finally announce most forcibly 'in a good light' (Beard, 1991).

- We tend too readily to pass off malaise and fever to influenza, yet it could represent another infectious disease either in the prodromal phase or in its full clinical development, or a more sinister disease such as infective endocarditis.

Time-clock fever: each day at 4 pm

Les J, a 53-year-old builder, was referred for a mitral valve replacement for long-standing mitral stenosis. His postoperative course had been uncomplicated and he was discharged from hospital on the 14th postoperative day. He was convalescing at home when, on the 23rd postoperative day, he suddenly developed fever with chills, headache, and muscle and joint pains. He did not complain of a sore throat or respiratory symptoms. On examination his temperature was 38.5 °C, pulse 102 and irregular (atrial fibrillation), BP 120/70 and respiratory rate 22/minute. The other abnormalities were bilateral basal crepitations, mild ankle oedema, cervical lymphadenopathy and hepatomegaly. His urine had a trace of protein, blood and bilirubin. His medication was digoxin, frusemide, potassium chloride and warfarin.

Following the home visit I admitted him to hospital with the provisional diagnosis of bacterial endocarditis (foremost), infectious mononucleosis (IM) or a urinary infection. He had undergone perfusion with fresh whole blood during surgery and thus blood-transmitted infections such as IM, hepatitis A or B, malaria and brucellosis were considered possible. I took blood for routine examination, culture, heterophil antibodies and liver function tests. A mid-stream urine sample (MSU) was sent for microscopy and culture.

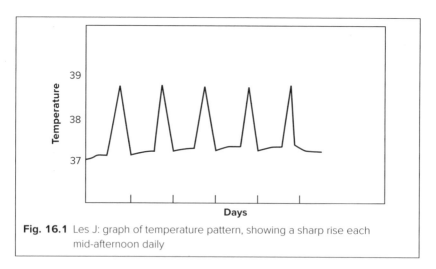

Fig. 16.1 Les J: graph of temperature pattern, showing a sharp rise each mid-afternoon daily

His fever and other symptoms settled spontaneously after four hours and on review the following day he said he felt well and would like to go home. However, at precisely 4 pm the fever returned and it subsequently returned at 4 pm each day. His temperature would then return to 37.2 °C within four to six hours (Figure 16.1).

Diagnosis and outcome

The results of Les J's investigations were as follows:

Hb (Haemoglobin) 14 g/L (normal indices)

WCC 12 600 lymphocytosis, many abnormal lymphocytes

MSU—many RBCs (red blood cells): normal culture

Sputum culture—no pathogens isolated

Chest X-ray—mild interstitial oedema, venous congestion

ECG—atrial fibrillation, incomplete RBBB (right bundle branch block), no evidence of ischaemia

IM screening test—negative, no heterophil antibodies

Blood culture—no growth after six days

Liver function tests—abnormal (moderate elevation of enzymes)

I realised that isolating a bacterial organism on blood culture would prove difficult because of previous exposure to antibiotics for a chest infection.

I consulted with his cardiologist who suggested arranging serial antibody titres for cytomegalovirus.

Les had acquired cytomegalovirus infection from the blood transfusion and his fever continued to spike in the mid-afternoon each day for about three weeks. There was no specific treatment. He eventually settled and had no long-term effects from the extraordinary infection.

DISCUSSION AND LESSONS LEARNED

- Unfamiliarity with uncommon infections can be confusing. Next time around it should be easier to recognise the fever patterns.
- It is still important to consider foremost the common or serious causes of cardiac postoperative fever such as bacterial endocarditis or urinary tract infection.
- Previous or current administration of antibiotics can mask any responsible bacterial organism, making isolation on culture difficult, if not impossible. Hence antibiotics should be used judiciously in these patients.
- Taking anticoagulants can cause red blood cells to appear in the urine and give the impression of urinary infection.
- Cytomegalovirus infection should be suspected on clinical grounds, especially in patients who have undergone open-heart surgery or renal transplantation. It causes a febrile illness (resembling glandular fever), which often manifests as quotidian intermittent fever, spiking to a maximum in the mid-afternoon and falling to normal each day. There is usually a relative lymphocytosis with atypical lymphocytes (similar to IM) but the heterophil antibody test is negative. Liver function tests are often abnormal. Generalised lymphadenopathy and hepatomegaly are typical. Specific diagnosis can be made by demonstrating rising antibody titres— four-fold increase. PCR (polymerase chain reaction) testing can now be used. The virus can be isolated from the urine and blood.
- It requires considerable skill and reassurance to convince patients to 'sweat it out' for up to six weeks of daily fevers, without specific medication.

Pyrexia in an Asian migrant

An 18-year-old migrant from an Asian country presented with a five-day history of fever, malaise and muscle aching; the onset coincided with his arrival in Australia. The man was previously fit and came from a professional family. He was said to be immunised against cholera and typhoid although it was not compulsory in his former country. There were no physical abnormalities on examination, apart from a temperature of 37.5 °C. He was told to rest and return if his symptoms persisted or worsened.

He presented a week later with a high fever, rigors, constipation and a slight cough. He appeared to be very ill, but apart from a temperature of 40 °C and cervical lymphadenopathy, the physical examination proved normal. His pulse rate was 80 beats per minute. The diagnosis was pyrexia of unknown origin (PUO).

The following tests were ordered: full blood examination; ESR; blood sugar, sodium, potassium, urea and creatinine; liver function tests; microscopy and culture of urine; and blood cultures. Blood film showed abnormalities: a marked left shift in polymorphs with toxic granulation; and the blood culture was positive, with Gram-negative rods, identified as *Escherichia coli*.

On clinical review the patient's condition was unchanged. A diagnosis of septicaemia was made and he was admitted to hospital.

Progress in hospital

The patient was treated with intravenous ampicillin, and blood cultures were repeated. His chest X-ray was normal. The spiking fever and rigors continued; pulse dissociation was observed (pulse did not increase when temperature rose). A soft systolic murmur was heard.

On the 16th day of his illness diarrhoea suddenly developed, after persistent constipation.

The revised diagnosis

The second set of blood cultures from the hospital laboratory confirmed the presence of Gram-negative rod organisms sensitive to all antibiotics.

After a consultant's opinion, intravenous gentamicin was started. However, further laboratory reports identified the organism as *Salmonella* Typhi and serological tests showed a raised titre for *S.* Typhi. A definitive diagnosis of typhoid fever was made and chloramphenicol 1.6 g was given intravenously every six hours.

The patient began to improve clinically, despite a drop in systolic blood pressure to 80 or 90 mm Hg. He was observed carefully for the serious complication of bowel perforation during the convalescent stage but (at the time of writing) is gradually improving. His present low-residue diet is high in protein and calories, with a small fluid intake. Forbidden are milk products, yeast foods, cold and effervescent drinks, and copious fluids. Encouraged are fish and boiled rice and potatoes.

DISCUSSION AND LESSONS LEARNED

- Laboratories can make mistakes. The first interpretation mistook the *S.* Typhi organisms for *E. coli*—both Gram-negative rods. However, *E. coli* ferments lactose and forms indole in peptone broth.
- Immunisation does not guarantee immunity from disease.
- Serious uncommon diseases alien to Australia should be suspected in overseas visitors with pyrexia of unknown origin.
- First-line treatment for typhoid acquired in the Indian sub-continent or Southeast Asia is now azithromycin.

Fever from the tropics

Initial consultation

A 42-year-old tractor mechanic presented with a four-day history of anorexia, malaise, non-specific joint and muscle pain, and fever. A previously fit man, he had just returned from 12 months working in rural Indonesia, Papua New Guinea and the Solomon Islands. He was known to be vaccinated against tetanus, polio and typhoid, and had been taking weekly antimalaria prophylaxis (chloroquine and Maloprim) until his return to Australia, three days previously.

Clinical examination was normal apart from his temperature of 38.1 °C. A full blood count was normal. The provisional diagnosis was influenza and he was instructed to rest and take paracetamol.

Subsequent consultation

The patient returned three days later complaining that his symptoms had not improved and he had now developed vomiting and mild diarrhoea. Examination confirmed the pyrexia (38.6 °C) and scleral jaundice was noted. A provisional diagnosis of viral hepatitis was made and investigations to confirm this diagnosis were arranged.

On review, the full blood count was again normal, but liver function tests confirmed hepatic dysfunction with elevated levels of bilirubin and hepatic transaminase. However, serology for hepatitis A and B was negative.

Progress

The patient was admitted to hospital where his unremitting fever was confirmed and his jaundice deepened. The diagnosis of malaria was considered and thick blood films were arranged. The first film was negative but the second, taken six hours later, demonstrated the presence of malarial parasites.

A careful and prolonged search of a concomitant thin blood film confirmed the diagnosis of *Plasmodium falciparum* malaria. The patient was treated with oral quinine, and over the subsequent days all symptoms and signs resolved.

The patient remained well and monthly blood films for the next three months failed to detect asexual parasitic stages.

DISCUSSION AND LESSONS LEARNED

- Australia is malaria free, but each year an increasing number of malaria cases, the majority due to *Plasmodium vivax*, are recorded. Most are acquired in the south-west Pacific region (Papua New Guinea, Vanuatu,

Solomon Islands) where *P. falciparum* malaria is both prevalent and widespread.

- While chloroquine and Maloprim prophylaxis were appropriate for this patient, no prophylactic regimen can guarantee total protection. The diagnosis of malaria should be entertained in all patients presenting with pyrexia on returning from an area where malaria is endemic.
- None of the symptoms and signs of malaria is specific. Unremitting temperature, rather than classic periodicity, is not uncommon. Malaria is a great mimic of other diseases, in particular influenza and viral hepatitis.
- Definitive diagnosis of malaria depends on microscopic determination of parasites in the peripheral blood film. A thick blood film is superior in making the diagnosis, because it concentrates red cells by a factor of 20 to 40 times. This is particularly important in patients with low levels of parasitaemia, especially those who have taken antimalarial therapy. Thick films are not routinely performed during full blood counts, unless the clinician indicates that malaria is a diagnostic possibility.

Beware the sweats by night

Leaving the comforting arms of the major teaching hospitals and stepping out into the wide, relatively unprotected world of general practice offers a frightening, yet exciting challenge for the emerging young doctor.

Each time the door to the consulting room opens, I wonder what problem lurks behind the disguise of the patient's symptoms. Will I flippantly say, 'It's just a virus going around', or will I read too hard between the lines, hoping I won't miss a rare case of 'X disease'. I have learned that being on guard is the only way of finding the happy medium and maintaining a sane equilibrium.

Two patients I saw within a month demonstrate just how unpredictable and exciting general practice can be for the young 'player'.

Nothing seemed amiss

Mrs S, a 68-year-old woman, presented one busy Monday morning with a dry irritating cough that she had had on and off for three months. She was rather anxious and nervously cleared her throat several times during the consultation.

Nothing seemed amiss on clinical examination, except that she appeared to be the type of person who 'overreacts' to simple everyday symptoms. I reassured her it was probably a 'post-viral cough', prescribed some cough mixture and ushered her to the door. As she turned to go, she off-handedly mentioned her troublesome sweats at night—'probably my hot flushes'. I nodded agreement and asked her to return next week.

On her next visit she was concerned that her cough was no better, and she was getting worn out from her dreadful hot flushes at night. There before me, on closer examination, was a large firm lump in her right axilla. My heart sank. Biopsy two days later confirmed Hodgkin lymphoma. CT scan confirmed mediastinal disease, thus her respiratory symptoms. Not all night sweats are hot flushes.

A lethargic geologist

Mr A, a pleasant 61-year-old retired geologist, presented with a three-week history of night sweats. He had recently returned from field work in caves near Cairns. His only other complaints were of some myalgia and lethargy, and he jokingly remarked how, while he was exploring a cave, a bat had scratched his face. On examination, he simply did not look well, but no concrete signs of disease could be found. The usual blood tests for PUO were ordered, as was a chest X-ray. The films showed multiple rounded opacities throughout both lung fields. Excitement and disbelief welled up inside me. The local respiratory physician confirmed he had acute histoplasmosis, often a self-limiting flu-like illness caused by inhalation of bat droppings laden with the fungus.

DISCUSSION AND LESSONS LEARNED

- So here, in the short space of a month, two patients presented with night sweats, both with rare causes. So easily could I have missed the diagnoses. I was assured by those around me that time and experience would allow the warning signals to develop. At least on most occasions.
- General practice is full of surprises and challenges. I found those first few months of general practice difficult, but also very rewarding.
- No . . . not everything is the flu or hot flushes!

The febrile Filipino bride

One Sunday I was asked to visit a 22-year-old woman who was very ill and unable to attend the surgery. I entered the bedroom on a very hot day to find a very apprehensive, shy woman of Asian heritage well rugged up in a warm water bed shaking with rigors. Her Australian-born husband explained that they had only arrived in the country three days previously, after being married in Manila the previous week. Ophelia did not communicate well and was most reluctant to be examined. She indicated that her symptoms were fever, chills, headache, backache and nausea. My provisional diagnosis, of course, was malaria. Not much doubt about it. Fortunately, I organised the appropriate screening tests.

Diagnosis

A phone call from the pathology laboratory the same evening revealed the cause. The urine was full of pus cells, bacteria and some red blood cells. The blood film seemed normal. The diagnosis was obvious—honeymoon cystitis/pyelitis.

DISCUSSION AND LESSONS LEARNED

- Funny how *Escherichia coli* travels across continents and is not mosquito-borne!

- Amazing how often it is a cause of pyrexia and certainly the commonest cause of rigors in the author's experience. Fooled again by the old urinary infection trap.
- It is important to think of common causes first and foremost.

Keeping an open mind

It was early Saturday afternoon—the morning surgery was over and the potentially long afternoon was beginning. The phone rang and a male voice spoke. 'My wife has been vomiting all morning—can you come?' As I was not busy at the time I was pleased to say that I could come soon. I grabbed some Maxolon on my way out, imagining that the problem would be one of viral gastroenteritis.

On arrival I found a woman aged in her 40s lying on the couch looking pale but certainly in keeping with the probable diagnosis. She gave a history of going to bed quite well but waking at her usual time with overwhelming nausea, vomiting and profuse watery diarrhoea. This had continued all morning. As she was not known at the practice, I enquired about her history as I examined her. She stated that she was well apart from some arthritis. Her medication consisted of prednisolone, methotrexate and penicillamine. She was under the care of a local rheumatologist. On examination she was pale and sweaty. Her pulse was fast and weak (120). Chest and abdominal examination were unremarkable. Her blood pressure was almost unrecordable—about 30 mm Hg systolic—which came as an unexpected surprise. A similar reading was obtained on the opposite limb. Her temperature was 39.5 °C (*per axilla*). She was clinically septic. The seriousness of the situation was conveyed to her husband. An ambulance was rung and an intravenous line quickly inserted.

Two hours later when I rang to check her condition, she was in intensive care with the provisional diagnosis of septic shock requiring intravenous antibiotics and inotropes to maintain her blood pressure. Subsequent investigations revealed a gram-negative septicaemia related to a urinary tract infection. No doubt her immunosuppressive medication had contributed to this event.

DISCUSSION AND LESSONS LEARNED

- This case reinforced my strategy to *always* ask a new patient for a full history and present medications. Many times I have been surprised by the answers I receive about these from patients who on initial impression look well.
- It is important to *always* examine the patient as fully as possible. In this case had I not checked her blood pressure it is possible that the gravity of her situation may not have been realised.
- *Always* keep an open mind on possible diagnoses—common things occur commonly, but not always.

A truly cryptic infection

Patrick, a 30-year-old Indigenous man, presented with a seven-day history of constant and increasing low thoracic back pain with two days of paraesthesia in the right groin. The constant pain especially night pain rang 'alarm bells'. What must not be missed? Checklist: VIC-Vascular, Infection or Cancer?

I firmly percussed his spine and there was definite tenderness over T12. His temperature was 37.6 °C (quite significant for a morning reading). He did have a furuncle in his groin and I suspected he was an intravenous drug user although he denied it.

I made the brave provisional diagnosis of epidural (or extradural) abscess, took blood for culture, ordered a plain X-ray (the desirable MRI scan was unavailable to us) and commenced him on flucloxacillin. The blood culture was positive for *Staphylococcus aureus* sensitive to flucloxacillin. Happily, Patrick did well.

DISCUSSION AND LESSONS LEARNED

- This uncommon focal infection of the CNS (central nervous system) can be extremely difficult to diagnose so an index of suspicion is required to consider a spinal epidural or subdural abscess. Late diagnosis may leave the patient with permanent and severe neurological disability.
- The typical clinical features of spinal epidural abscess include back pain and tenderness, fever, radiating root pain, paraesthesia and paraplegia. Most spinal epidural abscesses are thought to arise from the haematogenous spread of bacteria.
- Patrick was febrile, which made for an easier diagnosis, but fever may be absent. In about one third of cases the abscess may arise spontaneously but we must think of it for back pain following a post-subdural or epidural anaesthetic block.

The country dunny syndrome or 'rural flu'

Young country lads and perhaps even older men often use colourful phrases to express their feelings of disease. I recall that many adolescents use the ugly term 's***house' to express their feelings when seriously sick. Some would use the more acceptable term (to their doctor) 'country dunny'. During my term in rural practice it was not uncommon for a young fellow, often feeling awkward about visiting the doctor, to say 'I feel s***house, Doc' in response to the opening question about how they felt. This of course is not confined to rural males. Invariably they had influenza or a more virulent upper respiratory infection. However, one had to be cautious rather than dismissing this as an 'easy' management issue. Sometimes the problem was Epstein–Barr mononucleosis or even a more sinister infection.

The case of William

William was a robust 21-year-old man who worked on his father's dairy farm. The farm also carried beef cattle and a few sheep. He presented with a febrile illness plus sweating, myalgia, headache, weakness and arthralgia. The illness was in the context of an influenza pandemic and I made the provisional diagnosis of influenza and advised symptomatic treatment and asked him to let me know if he was not making progress or became worse. About four weeks later his mother said that she was most concerned about William, who was lethargic and moping around the farm. He would get episodes of fever that would subside after a few days and then return. This made me think about a younger woman who had recently been diagnosed with Hodgkin disease associated with relapsing fever. I organised to review him and I found that he certainly did not look well. He said that he felt depressed and wondered if he had chronic fatigue syndrome. He did confirm that he had recurrent fever at night followed by profuse sweating in the morning and then days of absence of fever. The possibility of a zoonosis occurred to me especially with the undulant fever pattern. I asked if he drank fresh milk. 'Yes—unpasteurised milk.'

Tests confirmed that he did have brucellosis.

DISCUSSION AND LESSONS LEARNED

- Occupational infectious diseases always have to be considered in patients presenting with an atypical febrile illness, especially atypical pneumonia.
- William was only one of only two cases of brucellosis (undulant fever) that the author encountered in the many years associated with the dairy industry, and that was a long time ago.

Neurological dilemmas

The bothered and bewildered amnesic patient

Harry, a 62-year-old man with a history of hypertension and anxiety, presented one evening because of the acute onset of an amnesic episode. He had driven to collect his two grandchildren from school that afternoon. The children reported that their grandfather appeared his usual self except that he was unable to find his way home. He drove around the neighbourhood for about three hours before eventually locating his house with the help of the children. Upon returning home his family found him confused and unable to remember the events. I found him perplexed and repeatedly asking where he was and how he came to be there. The children said that his driving seemed normal. Harry could not give an account of the day's events nor could he remember getting up that morning. He could not recall significant recent events such as an overseas holiday. Physical examination was normal.

I had not encountered this amnesic syndrome before so I phoned a consultant neurologist who informed me that it was probably a classic case of transient global amnesia and that the amnesic state should resolve completely, leaving only a memory gap for events that occurred during the episode.

I have subsequently encountered two other episodes over the years, including that of a 67-year-old GP friend who found himself confused at an end-of-line suburban railway station on a line quite remote from his usual route home. The initial experience with Harry was a great help in understanding the disorder and thus helped to confidently counsel subsequent patients.

DISCUSSION AND LESSON LEARNED

Sometimes we are consulted for a problem that is foreign to our current state of medical knowledge. For me it is often a neurological problem such as transient global amnesia. I find that the best strategy is to contact a helpful consultant or GP colleague (immediately if possible) and talk through the problem.

All locked in

Many years ago, a worried friend contacted me after a flight from London to explain that she had a sudden terrifying experience when she could not speak or use her arms. No one came to her aid because she appeared to be asleep and could not rouse her husband or use the call button. She said that the symptoms gradually abated over the next 15 minutes or so and she felt reasonably normal now. It occurred to me that this was a transient ischaemic attack (TIA) causing the 'locked-in syndrome'; I organised an urgent visit to a neurological unit. Subsequently Bernie has been taking low-dose aspirin for 17 years without any further cerebrovascular incidents.

DISCUSSION AND LESSONS LEARNED

- The so-called 'locked-in syndrome' is dramatic and of particular concern because it affects the brain stem. The more dramatic stroke is a catastrophe for the patient and their family, and popular magazines describe real-life stories about patients who are unable to speak or use their limbs but who are conscious and aware of their predicament. However, they can communicate with their eyes in response to commands and we should consider this in mute paralysed patients.
- Such an episode reinforces the importance of the think FAST strategy for TIAs and stroke: namely Face, Arms, Speech and Time (act within three hours and refer to a stroke unit) but don't give aspirin at this stage.

- Furthermore, there is a high risk that a patient presenting with a TIA will proceed to have a stroke, particularly in the first six months.
- One of the more common TIAs that we encounter is amaurosis fugax which is sudden transient loss of vision in one eye following an embolus originating in the ipsilateral carotid artery.

A breathtaking episode of post-flu fatigue

Jenny M, aged 16, a bright schoolgirl and active sportsgirl, was brought along with her somewhat overbearing and overprotective father because she was feeling 'weak in the arms', especially around the right arm and wrist, where she described a tingling sensation that had been there for the past 24 hours.

Her recent history was that of a mild febrile illness 'rather like the flu' a few days beforehand and several hard games of tennis in a tournament that finished the previous day. 'Doctor—you tell her—she's overdoing it. All this activity even with the flu. She's still a growing girl.'

Jenny complained also of headache, nausea and an aching jaw as well as the feeling of weakness in her right arm, which I attributed to soreness following her sporting overload and her viral infection. Reflex testing was equivocal and sensation normal. A tentative diagnosis of post-influenzal weakness aggravated by overuse was made, and father and daughter were reassured. I did wonder about the possibility of cervical spondylosis or carpal tunnel syndrome but thought that her relative youth was against these diagnoses.

Two days later her father rang to inform me that Jenny was confined to bed, her legs were now weak and she was unable to walk properly. 'Is it anything to worry about?'

The home visit

'Yes, it is something to worry about,' I thought, with that sickly feeling that a serious neurological or infectious disorder had been overlooked. Jenny was indeed in trouble. The change was quite dramatic—two days previously she walked into my surgery looking fit but now she was very weak in all limbs with obvious motor weakness and loss of reflexes. She was also having trouble breathing: 'Taking a normal deep breath seems impossible'. I tested her peak flow and it was markedly reduced.

Diagnosis and outcome

Jenny was suffering from Guillain–Barré syndrome (acute post-infective polyneuritis) with respiratory involvement. She was admitted to hospital where she eventually received assisted ventilation for a few days without developing complete paralysis. She made a complete recovery.

DISCUSSION AND LESSONS LEARNED

- Guillain–Barré syndrome, although rare (12 cases per million per year), can catch us by surprise especially if we get sidetracked by focusing on common causes such as fatigue from overuse or influenza. Diagnosis in the early stages is obviously important.
- Neurological-type symptoms following a viral infection should demand considerable respect and careful examination. In over two-thirds, a viral infection precedes the onset of neuropathy by one to three weeks.

Real headaches

Case 1

One Sunday afternoon I was startled by the sound of a car hurriedly charging into my driveway and then the almost inhuman sound of a strange, high-pitched wailing. A young woman was in the car in a stuporous state, unable to communicate normally and emitting a haunting, agonised, loud wail. According to her husband they were driving along, enjoying the drive through the hills, when she suddenly grabbed her head and screamed out. Examining this hitherto healthy woman in a car was difficult but I noted that her neck was virtually rigid. We drove her to hospital where I performed a lumbar puncture—evenly blood-stained cerebrospinal fluid (CSF). Subarachnoid haemorrhage! She was transferred to a city hospital and survived, but with a neurological deficit.

Case 2

One morning I was called urgently to the home of a 43-year-old woman with a long-standing history of severe migraine. She was dead in bed. The previous evening she had developed a sudden severe headache with associated vomiting after getting into bed. Her husband called the locum service. The headache had eased considerably when a young doctor eventually arrived to examine her. He said that she was experiencing a particularly severe migraine attack and gave her an injection of morphine, which helped considerably and she went to sleep around 10.30 pm—never to awaken.

DISCUSSION AND LESSONS LEARNED

- The subarachnoid haemorrhage, especially with milder cases, can be a very elusive diagnosis, particularly in the absence of neck stiffness and neurological changes. A good working rule is: 'A sudden headache represents a subarachnoid haemorrhage until proved otherwise'.
- Patients with a history of severe migraine present a special problem when they develop the sudden headache of subarachnoid haemorrhage.
- Subarachnoid haemorrhage is occasionally overlooked, mainly because it is not considered in the differential diagnosis (especially if a milder form). About one-third of patients experience a 'sentinel' headache (a warning leak) in the hours to days before the major bleed. Neck stiffness or a positive Kernig's sign, drowsiness, a persistent neurological deficit or a particularly severe and protracted headache should raise suspicion. If in doubt, a CT head scan will usually establish the diagnosis, or if this does not, a lumbar puncture will. A follow-up visit within 12 or 24 hours is wise when there is some lingering doubt. Early referral for coiling or clipping the

offending aneurysm is vital, because the better the patient's condition the higher the chance of complete recovery after surgery.

- Visiting patients late at night can cloud one's judgement. A darkened room combined with 'darkened' feelings from a tired doctor represents a suboptimal 'office' for consultation. We need to discipline ourselves not to let these adverse factors affect our professionalism.

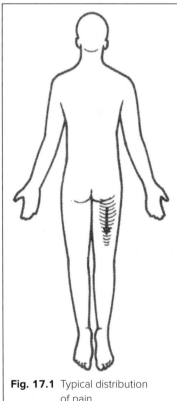

Fig. 17.1 Typical distribution of pain

Hip-pocket nerve syndrome

Andy P, aged 54, presented with a 12-month history of pain in his right thigh. The pain was gradually getting worse to the point where Andy was considering quitting driving his taxi. He claimed that the pain started at 'the bone' of the buttock and extended down the back of his thigh to the knee (Figure 17.1). It was aggravated by sitting, relieved by standing and did not bother him at night. There was no inflammatory component to the pain in that it was eased by rest and was absent on waking in the morning. Furthermore, the history did not suggest claudication as a cause.

The only abnormal finding on physical examination was tenderness over the sciatic nerve at the level of the ischial tuberosity. Examination of the lumbosacral spine and regional nervous system was normal. The slump test for dural irritation was negative.

The cause of his sciatica, which is invariably of spinal origin, was puzzling and so an X-ray of his lumbosacral spine was ordered. This was normal. He continued to complain bitterly of the ache and so he was ordered a CT scan, which was also normal.

Diagnosis and outcome

On review I pondered the possible cause and considered whether pressure from a wallet in his hip pocket could be the cause. After all, he was constantly sitting as part of his occupation. I asked to inspect his wallet, which was 'hard and bulky' and contained 12 plastic credit cards. He returned three weeks after a trial of removing the wallet from his right hip pocket to explain that his pain had gradually disappeared.

DISCUSSION AND LESSONS LEARNED

- Andy's problem was simply solved by the powers of observation and common sense. We so often fail to look for the obvious mechanical reason for an unusual presentation.
- If a man presents with right-sided (or maybe even left-sided) sciatica, especially confined to the buttock and upper thigh (without local back pain), one should always consider the possibility of pressure on the sciatic nerve from a wallet or other hard object in the hip pocket.

Fits and funny turns: the case of Terryanne

Terryanne, a 23-year-old housewife, is an epileptic. At our first consultation I found she was being treated with phenytoin and phenobarbitone in dosages that had been juggled over the past two years by the local hospital and other practitioners. Despite this supervision, her clinical equilibrium was fragile. At times she exhibited a variety of neurological symptoms: dizziness, ataxia, paraesthesiae, slurred speech, hyperactivity and 'funny turns'.

I started a regular check of her phenytoin and phenobarbitone blood levels. Despite her insistence that she always took her tablets exactly as prescribed,

Terryanne's blood levels fluctuated above and below the normal limits. Her symptoms indicated high or 'toxic' levels of phenytoin.

Factors that could be responsible for these fluctuations in her blood levels

- Poor compliance (despite her claims to the contrary).
- Confusion caused by the drugs.
- Alcohol and other drugs of self-abuse such as marijuana.
- Drug interactions.

Phenytoin has been described as the most 'capricious' drug in the doctor's pharmacopoeia, with the potential to react adversely with almost any substance.

Drugs that interfere with metabolism and cause a drop in serum levels include other anticonvulsants (such as phenobarbitone, carbamazepine and clonazepam), alcohol and folic acid. Drugs that raise the serum level include oral anticoagulants, diazepam, propranolol, frusemide, phenothiazines, phenylbutazone, disulfiram and isoniazid.

After checking the drug interaction guide I decided to discontinue phenobarbitone and substitute primidone, which was not implicated. However, the same problems continued. Often her husband would phone me late in the evening with the information that Terryanne was having a 'funny turn'—acting strangely—and occasionally that she was very agitated.

I suspected alcohol abuse and conducted an investigation befitting Sherlock Holmes, but it drew a blank: alcohol definitely was not involved. I continued probing and during a consultation I learned she had been taking phentermine, prescribed some years ago for weight reduction. I had the answer at last.

Diagnosis and outcome

Terryanne had developed psychological and physiological dependence on the drug. She had stockpiled it, taking it for anxiety, stress or any manner of 'disease' for several days until she felt 'normal'. Using diazepam as a temporary substitute I weaned her off the phentermine; she does not have strange turns or symptoms any more. Two EEGs have shown normal activity, and primidone has been stopped.

DISCUSSION AND LESSONS LEARNED

- The hazards of drug interactions cannot be overemphasised. If clinical equilibrium has not been established, the general practitioner has to search beyond the history for the influence of other drugs, especially alcohol. In this case phentermine, a central nervous system (CNS) stimulant, retarded the metabolism of phenytoin.
- When there is difficulty in stabilising a patient on drug therapy, blood levels of the prescribed substance should be checked and monitored.

Tremors and shock waves

Peter, a 30-year-old computer technician from Sydney, first presented to me for another opinion about his problem of 'the shakes' and 'funny speech'. For the past five years he had noted the gradual onset of shaking of his hands, especially when doing things such as writing or picking up a cup of tea. Over this time his writing had become a real problem and he was prone to tumble when walking, especially walking downhill.

His speech was also a problem and his family and friends remarked on how slow and deliberate it had become. Apart from these neurological symptoms he felt quite well. He had consulted three other doctors, including a neurologist, over the previous three years and they could not diagnose his disorder. His family doctor thought he had early Parkinson's disease. He was not taking any drugs—prescribed or self-administered.

On examination, he had a healthy appearance, an intention-type tremor and mild dysarthria. There was some rigidity of his upper limbs.

The problem confused me, and so I referred Peter to another neurologist for diagnosis and management. He said that he was also puzzled and arranged magnetic resonance imaging (MRI) of Peter's brain. This test indicated the presence of demyelination in the area of the basal ganglia. The consultant concluded that he had an 'exaggerated essential tremor' and no treatment was warranted.

Other developments in siblings

On review the usual calm and laconic Peter claimed to be very angry with the medical professional for not giving him a satisfactory explanation for the slowly worsening problem and for indulging themselves in an investigation that left him almost $1000 out of pocket. I tried to support him as best I could, and after a year or so he contacted me to say that his 19-year-old sister had been admitted to hospital in Adelaide because of 'severe swelling of her body'. She was diagnosed as having cirrhosis of the liver. Incredibly, within a few weeks his 26-year-old brother was considered to have a liver disorder.

Diagnosis and outcome

It was now obvious that Peter and his siblings suffered from the familial disorder of Wilson's disease (hepatolenticular degeneration). It is an autosomal recessive disorder in which the inherited metabolic defect is associated with the deposition of copper in the liver or central nervous system, or both.

On review we observed the greenish-brown corneal pigmentation (Kayser–Fleischer ring) even with the naked eye, and it was quite outstanding with slit-lamp examination.

Peter has responded extremely well to treatment with penicillamine. His tremor and dysarthria have improved dramatically, but his corneal copper deposits remind us of how we initially 'missed the boat'. His liver function is good, but his younger siblings still have liver problems. He continues to complain *ad nauseam* about the lost $1000!

DISCUSSION AND LESSONS LEARNED

- Although rarely encountered, disorders such as Wilson's disease are difficult to diagnose, and it is important to aggressively pursue apparent genuine neurological symptoms, especially in the younger patient.
- It is important to explain the costs of and reasons for investigations and procedures, especially where considerable expenses are involved.

- If Wilson's disease is suspected the patient should have an ocular slit-lamp examination, a check on serum ceruloplasmin levels (low in 95 per cent of patients) and a liver biopsy. Early diagnosis and treatment mean a better prognosis.

Two 'fishy' tales

Case 1: the child who 'died'

A 2-year-old Vietnamese girl presented in dramatic circumstances to the emergency department of a country hospital when I was on duty. She was apnoeic and required manual ventilation by the ambulance officers. They claimed that they went on a call expecting to find a pregnant woman in labour, but instead they found a young Vietnamese woman with her daughter 'asleep' in her arms. They noticed that the child was not breathing and thought she was dead, but she had a full pulse. They promptly began artificial ventilation, her colour improved and she remained in a stable condition during the ambulance trip.

On examination in casualty she had a normal colour, a full bounding pulse, normal heart sounds and blood pressure—but no spontaneous respiration. Neurological assessment revealed generalised hypotonia, areflexia (including plantar reflex), fixed dilated pupils and no response to painful stimuli. There were no other abnormal findings in any other system and no evidence of injury. A blood glucose estimation (glucometer) was 6 mmol/L.

The child was promptly intubated and cardiac monitored, and an intravenous line was inserted.

The language barrier made it difficult to obtain an accurate history. However, I was able to ascertain that shortly after eating lunch the child staggered about as though 'drunk' and eventually fell to the floor and stopped breathing.

Diagnosis

My initial diagnostic hypotheses included aspiration or an intracerebral catastrophe, but I realised that the clinical information did not support this reasoning. On further questioning of the relatives I learned that for lunch the family had eaten a fish the father had caught off the pier of a Victorian coastal town.

Revised diagnosis

I diagnosed tetrodotoxic fish poisoning due to eating a toadfish ('toadie'). These poisonous fish are found around the coast of Australia. A quick reference to a text on toxic marine animals (Sutherland, 1983) provided information that the poisoning is characterised by progressive ataxia leading to respiratory paralysis, making it appear that the patient is dead. This did not explain why the parents were spared. Since the toxin is reported to concentrate in the liver and ovaries and only in small amounts in muscle, I considered that the child was served the offal and the parents ate the flesh.

Epilogue

The child was transferred to the intensive care ward of the Royal Children's Hospital, Melbourne, where she made a full recovery after three days. The prognosis for respiratory arrest in children is apparently excellent.

In Japan the toadfish (fugu) is a delicacy, but it can only be prepared by specially licensed chefs who manage to remove most of the tetrodotoxin from the flesh, although the toxin cannot be removed by washing or by prolonged cooking. Apparently, part of the enjoyment of eating the fish is the tingling sensation felt on the tongue due to small amounts of the toxin. There are several deaths a year in Japan due to ingestion of this fish. Captain Cook almost died in 1774 after sampling a little of the roe and liver of a toadfish in New Caledonia.

Case 2: a 'tingling' experience

A 40-year-old businessman holidaying in Queensland presented with extreme weakness, exhaustion and strange 'numb' and 'tingling' sensations around his mouth and in his hands, following an episode of diarrhoea, abdominal pain and vomiting. He gave a fascinating history of how he and his two mates went on a fishing trip near Cairns where they caught some large Spanish mackerel. They said they experienced a strange, cold, tingling feeling in the hands while cleaning the fish.

Five hours after eating one of the fish all three developed what they considered to be a 'gastric' attack with diarrhoea and vomiting. After this settled the patient was aware of aching in the joints and muscles as well as the tingling sensations. He said he also experienced a strange burning painful feeling when his hands were placed in cold water. 'I can't go swimming in the sea, Doctor—it feels terrible.' On examination he was afebrile and no specific abnormality could be found.

On review two weeks later he still felt weak and anorexic. He had pruritus of the skin and mild tingling sensations that became worse when exposed to cold factors such as water or ice cream.

Diagnosis

The patient has ciguatera poisoning due to eating a fish containing ciguatoxin. The problem can occur in all tropical and subtropical sea water to 30° latitude. The differential diagnosis is bacterial food poisoning, but this produces the rapid onset of gastrointestinal symptoms without peripheral neurological effects.

DISCUSSION AND LESSONS LEARNED

- Toxic reactions to eating fish should be considered if patients exhibit unusual neurological symptoms and signs including 'tingling' sensations of the extremities and respiratory paralysis.
- Obviously people should be warned about eating toad or 'puffer' fish and should avoid eating large carnivorous fish in some tropical waters. Moray eels should never be eaten, nor should the viscera or gonads of any tropical fish.

A colleague with dementia—missing the clues

Ron was a 67-year-old respected medical colleague who presented for a second opinion. He had visited his own general practitioner who, after conducting a mental state examination, was convinced that he had

Alzheimer's disease. When Ron came in my first impression was that dementia was not immediately obvious but there was something unusual about his gait. His judgement and concentration had declined but he was reasonably functional in day-to-day activities. He was accompanied by his wife, who said that he was now somewhat disorganised, especially with decision making, organising his accounts and other financial affairs. There was no family history of dementia.

On examination he was physically well but his apraxic gait was a stand-out. It was unsteady and broad-based with small steps; he seemed to be glued to the floor. His wife described a problem with urinary incontinence which was deteriorating. Still the 'penny did not drop'. His Mini-Mental State Examination or Folstein test was 20, indicating probable mild dementia.

We assumed that Ron did have a neurological abnormality and dementia and referred him to a specialist in the area. He performed an MRI study and diagnosed Alzheimer's disease and commenced him on medication. He managed at home for 18 months and eventually was admitted to a nursing home for special care. Six months later he was being reviewed by a geriatrician who considered the possibility of normal pressure hydrocephalus which was confirmed by further MRI scanning and lumbar puncture.

Ron underwent ventriculo-peritoneal shunting which led to an amazing transformation in his health to almost normality for some months before deteriorating gradually.

DISCUSSION AND LESSONS LEARNED

- We learn our diagnostic triads yet can miss the connection, especially with an uncommon neurological condition. The *classic triad for normal pressure hydrocephalus-apraxic gait, incontinence and dementia* was there to consider but was overlooked. Neurology is a challenging discipline! As always the early diagnosis of a serious but treatable condition is a priority.
- The other message is to consider an underlying reason for the diagnosis or condition, even dementia.

Children and brain-teasers

Chapter
18

The little girl who loved red and blue Lego

Charlotte, aged 30 months, was brought by her mother to the clinic because she was concerned about her development which did not seem to match that of her older cousin. She seemed slow to talk and not interested in socialising with other children. She was also prone to temper tantrums. She was born prematurely at 35 weeks and had an Apgar score of 9. She walked at 12 months, had a good appetite, could activate electronic toys and games as well as make excellent Lego constructions. On examination, including a neurological examination, Charlotte was very healthy but was reluctant to engage with us. Although her general milestones were satisfactory we took cognisance of mother's concerns and arranged to review her in three months.

At review there were further concerns. She was still slow to talk, slow to toilet train and socialise. The director of the childcare centre was concerned about her tendency to play by herself and seek out a particular red toy and play with Lego particularly with red and blue blocks.

She got frustrated easily and fell to the floor when adults could not understand her wants and the temper tantrums were more dramatic. We still observed her poor eye contact; she tended to avoid looking at a person by directing her gaze elsewhere. She would not engage with relatives and strangers unless she wanted something. By now we suspected an autism spectrum disorder and referred her to a specialist paediatrician.

She diagnosed austism and recommended a multidisciplinary rehabilitation program with the emphasis on development of language and social skills.

DISCUSSION AND LESSONS LEARNED

- The diagnosis of behavioural developmental disorders in early childhood is not easy so early referral to a disability unit or specialist is advisable, especially as early intervention can produce significant improvement.
- Once again the principle of taking notice of parents' concerns and follow up for such a concern is important.

Beware the childhood dysplastic hip

We have all spent anxious moments wondering whether we have misdiagnosed developmental dysplasia of the hip and some of us have experienced nervous moments due to a delayed diagnosis.

Case 1

Dr Helen Fitzgerald writes about a full-term healthy baby girl who was checked by a paediatrician at birth and at six weeks post partum. No problems were identified. She attended at eight weeks for her first immunisation and was examined by another doctor who recorded a normal physical examination. At eight months she developed a febrile illness due to a urinary tract infection. The radiologist who performed a renal tract ultrasound contacted the practice to report that the baby's left hip was dislocated and the acetabulum and femoral head were abnormal.

Case 2

Dr David Howard records the case of a child of 17 months who was slotted into a hectic overbooked surgery despite not having a formal appointment. She was not walking normally, mostly on her tiptoes, and her mother believed she had been injured by her older brother who had a profound behavioural problem. An X-ray of the whole leg including the hip was ordered but the radiographer, after speaking to the mother, decided to X-ray the lower leg. The report was read but the fact that the hip was not imaged was overlooked. The dislocated hip was detected at a subsequent consultation but the diagnosis was unfortunately delayed beyond conservative correction.

Case 3

The author was asked to review a medico-legal case in which both the radiologist and general practitioner were sued for delayed diagnosis of a hip that required corrective surgery. The GP ordered a plain X-ray in the neonate and no abnormality was detected by the radiologist. An ultrasound examination was omitted but was positive at 15 months when the child presented with a limp. Of interest was the earlier opinion of the infant welfare nurse who advised of a positive Ortolani test. Both the GP and radiologist and their separate insurers were held responsible.

DISCUSSION AND LESSONS LEARNED

- Expect the unexpected. These infants had no risk factors such as family history or a breech delivery.
- Plain X-rays have no diagnostic value in the neonatal period but can be helpful after three months of age. Ultrasound examination is excellent especially up to three to four months.
- It is advisable to develop the routine of performing examination of the child's hip during routine presentation for review and immunisation. Take due recognition of any concerns of the mother and nurse.

Three children with blunt abdominal trauma

Case 1

Paul B, aged 7, came for assessment of his abdominal pain following a fall from his bicycle. Apparently, the handlebars struck his epigastric area as he catapulted over the bicycle. Initially he looked pale and uncomfortable but after two to three hours of observation he improved. He had tenderness over the area that was struck. As his observations were satisfactory we sent him home with an appointment for review the following morning.

On review, his condition was cause for concern. He looked pale, walked with extreme discomfort and had exquisite abdominal tenderness. Unfortunately, we did not have the luxury of CT scanning in those days. At laparotomy Paul was found to have retroperitoneal rupture of the duodenum from which he recovered after a stormy postoperative course.

Case 2

Simon J, aged 9, was playing football when he fell and struck his abdomen with his own elbow. He continued playing and went home but the pain became worse. On examination he was pale and uncomfortable and so we admitted him to hospital for observation. After an hour or so his blood pressure dropped, so urgent laparotomy was arranged. A ruptured spleen was repaired after haemostasis secured, with every effort being made to save the organ.

Case 3

One morning I was called urgently to the home of Jenny B, aged 13, who was found dead in bed. About 20 hours earlier she had been a passenger in a car accident in the city. After three hours' observation and despite persistent abdominal pain, she was discharged from the emergency department of the hospital. She returned home to her parents, who were concerned but thought they 'wouldn't bother me because she had been seen by the doctors and given the all clear'. Jenny died from the effects of a ruptured stomach.

DISCUSSION AND LESSONS LEARNED

- Children seem very prone to ruptured viscera from abdominal trauma, sometimes apparent trivial trauma. Retroperitoneal rupture of the duodenum was described many years ago as the 'handlebars injury'. Injury can often occur to the pancreas, liver, spleen and kidney.

- It is important to avoid laparotomy if possible, and nowadays the progress of these injuries can be monitored with ultrasound (especially for hollow organs) and CT scans (especially for solid organs).
- The spleen should be preserved if possible because patients without spleens are prone to fulminant infection with *Streptococcus pneumoniae* and other organisms.
- It is important to admit these injured children for observation for 24 hours.

Deadly little bugs in little children

Case 1

The mother of 3-year-old John B rang one lunchtime concerned that her son had developed a fever and cough, and she asked if he should be seen. About 30 minutes later, when I opened the door to a waiting room full of patients, I noted young John sitting on his mother's knee looking pale and floppy, breathing audibly through an open mouth making a snoring sound and drooling saliva from the corners of his mouth. I beckoned them into the office and noted that he was febrile (38.9 °C *per rectum*), had rib retraction and tachycardia.

John obviously had life-threatening acute epiglottitis. Apparently, his symptoms commenced only 90 minutes previously. We took him to our hospital and inserted an endotracheal tube in the operating theatre after clearing copious, tenacious mucus from the airway. We then connected him to the Bird's respirator for ventilation and commenced intravenous chloramphenicol. He had settled dramatically within 24 hours and we extubated him 48 hours after admission.

Case 2

The mother of 5-year-old Michael D rang to say that Michael had been sent home from school sick with the rather sudden onset of fever, headache, vomiting and a rash that had just appeared. 'Could be anything,' I thought. 'A viral exanthem? Measles?' But it didn't add up.

Seeing Michael caused the 'heartsink' feeling one occasionally gets when seeing a really sick child—prostrate, pale, whimpering, eyes following you around the room with only the head turning. On closer inspection he had a fine petechial rash on his shoulders and arms. Had to be meningococcal septicaemia. He was hastily transferred to hospital where blood was taken for culture and intravenous crystalline penicillin was given immediately. He recovered.

Case 3

Tom R, aged 6 months, was presented for a second time in two days because of fever, not feeding, general disinterest and vomiting. I noted a dramatic change in two days—he was very ill, flat and febrile. The striking observation was that his breathing was deep and rapid and his breath had a peculiar 'fruity' odour. I recalled, as a student, learning the differences between the hyperventilation of septicaemia and acidosis, and I thought that septicaemia was possible.

I immediately referred Tom to the children's hospital. By the time he arrived he was comatose. I could hardly believe that that beautiful, little boy had diabetic ketoacidosis as well as *E. coli* septicaemia. What a burden for him and his parents to carry. He survived to face a most uncertain future.

Case 4

Spiro P, aged 10 weeks, presented to the emergency department when I was a resident. He looked sick but, apart from this and a mild fever, I could find nothing wrong on clinical examination and was thinking of sending him home when a very experienced charge nurse said, 'Hey, that child's really sick; get the registrar in'. The registrar could find nothing abnormal and so the consultant was called in. 'Feel this,' he said, pointing to an enlarged liver. 'Listen to this abnormal heart.' The child had acute viral myocarditis and died six hours later in hospital.

DISCUSSION AND LESSONS LEARNED

- In the midst of all the simple, uncomplicated, viral, upper respiratory infections we have to be forever vigilant for that unexpected rare, but rapidly fatal, overwhelming infection. Such infections include acute epiglottitis (fortunately rare these days with *Haemophilus influenzae* type b vaccine given through the national immunisation program), meningococcal septicaemia, other septicaemias, acute bacterial meningitis, streptococcal infection in neonates and acute myocarditis.
- Once a lethal bacterial infection is diagnosed it is best to institute immediate antibiotic therapy after taking blood for culture. Waiting around for results before taking action is like playing Russian roulette with precious lives.
- As a general practitioner it is so important to be able to recognise the really sick children and then give them the attention they deserve. Such children lie quietly, are listless, pale and whimpering in contradistinction to the flushed, febrile, lustily crying and more robust children.

The scared little boy with insomnia

Steven, aged 7, was a bright, happy little boy until he developed an extraordinary and puzzling episode of insomnia which, much to our shame, was solved eventually by his teacher.

He presented to our group practice with his bemused mother who claimed that, suddenly, he would not and could not sleep. His parents would be startled at night by the eerie vision of Steven standing silent and motionless beside their bed. When not in his bed at night he would be found hiding under it or in his wardrobe.

His behaviour was normal otherwise, but his teacher reported his schoolwork had deteriorated and he was constantly falling asleep at his desk. On direct questioning Steven was shy and evasive, claiming nothing was worrying him. We considered it was a temporary phase of abnormal behaviour and advised conservative measures such as hot beverages, baths and exercises before retiring. This strategy failed and so Steven was prescribed hypnotics, initially in low dosage but finally in high dosage: to no avail.

His parents were convinced by now that he was psychologically disturbed. He was referred to a consultant who also failed to find a cause for the insomnia and advised long midnight jogs. The neighbourhood began to buzz with amusement at the sight of the tiny nocturnal jogger labouring beside the slow vehicle driven by his yawning father. This remarkable therapy did not work either.

At last, Steven's teacher had the bright idea of asking all the children to draw the thing that scared or worried them most, stipulating that it would be a 'make believe' picture. Looking at the drawing depicting two robbers stealing his moneybox as he slept (Figure 18.1), she tactfully confronted Steven, who admitted that his playmate had told him robbers would come one night, steal his moneybox and 'bash' him.

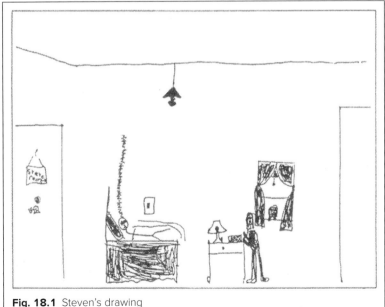

Fig. 18.1 Steven's drawing

The final chapter of this story saw a happy Steven perched on a bank counter watching his money being ceremoniously counted, deposited in a huge safe and exchanged for a bank book. Steven was convinced his precious money was safe and has slept normally ever since.

DISCUSSION AND LESSONS LEARNED

- Insomnia and nightmares can be the presenting feature of the disturbed child. One in ten children suffers from emotional disturbance; uncharacteristic presenting problems should not be dismissed lightly.
- Discussion of the problem can be difficult with disturbed children but asking them to 'draw a dream' (as suggested by Professor Bruce Tonge, 1983) is an excellent avenue to this important communication. (Professor Tonge believes that it is the royal road to the child's mental processes and the family doctor is ideally placed to use the technique.)

Bones and abdominal groans

This tale is about a 4-year-old girl called Claire who, full of life and inquisitiveness, is one of those delightful little girls who is very easy to relate to.

When Claire accompanied her mother and siblings to the surgery, she would invariably flit around the office asking a multitude of questions about various wall charts, models and instruments. Of particular attraction to her was a fully articulated skeleton, called 'Eric', which occupied a corner of the surgery (Figure 18.2). She was obsessed by it and would ask many questions.

'Was this a real person one day?'

'Yes.'

'Is he really dead?'

'Yes.'

'How did he die?'

My spontaneous reply was: 'He swallowed his bubble gum'.

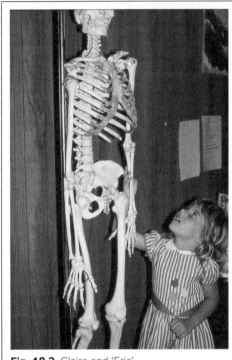

Fig. 18.2 Claire and 'Eric'

One evening I was requested to make a house call to Claire who was suffering from severe abdominal pain. I arrived to find her in considerable distress pointing to the umbilical area as the site of intense pain. She was sobbing and very emotional—quite out of character for the usually self-contained little girl. In fact my initial impression was that the presentation was bizarre, although not uncommon in children. The history was unrewarding— no anorexia or vomiting, no diarrhoea, no headache, no abnormal urinary symptoms and no recent history of stress, family upsets or other emotional problems. On examination there was vague tenderness around the periumbilical area but nothing specific. Her temperature and pulse were normal.

I reassured the parents that she did not appear to have a serious problem and I arranged for a visit early next morning at the hospital where we would take a urine specimen for microscopy and culture. Claire's parting words were: 'I don't want to die'—a very significant comment, which I failed to appreciate at the time.

On review she had slept well but had awoken sobbing and still complaining of pain. The urine was normal and I was even more convinced that the problem was functional. I asked again if she had eaten anything unusual in the past few days or swallowed any objects such as pins or coins.

'I swallowed my bubble gum,' Claire said sheepishly.

Beware comments to children

I had my fingers burned on another occasion when I told another inquisitive child that 'Eric' had once smoked more than 20 cigarettes a day. The child's unhappy grandfather then confronted me about my comments, because he had been reprimanded in no uncertain terms about his smoking habit.

DISCUSSION AND LESSONS LEARNED

- One has to be very diplomatic and cautious about comments concerning health to impressionable children.
- The non-medical person finds coping with the concept of a real skeleton somewhat overbearing. 'Eric' no longer stands in the surgery but in a museum's anatomy room. I found it very useful in my country practice with a high incidence of skeletal trauma, especially fractures and dislocations, for patient education.
- Functional abdominal pain in children is common in general practice and it is worthwhile exploring probable fears and emotional problems, such as marital disharmony in the home, child abuse, problems including bullying at school and perhaps indiscreet comments from their doctors!

Vertigo in children: two cases of 'scarlet face'

Case 1

Craig P, aged 9, was rushed dramatically into the surgery on 24 December 1982. His mother had left him at home about three hours previously and he had been perfectly well. She returned to find him in a stupor and staggering around the house. He was unable to give a coherent history. The mother claimed he had not been taking any drugs and there were no suspicious signs around the house.

Craig looked drowsy, stuporose and pale but would respond to basic commands. It was possible to ascertain that he had vertigo, a generalised headache and had vomited several times.

Significant findings on examination were:

- pulse 102; blood pressure 95/60; temperature 37 °C; respiratory rate 20/minute
- pupils dilated and reacting sluggishly to light
- bilateral nystagmus
- diplopia
- generalised muscular weakness (normal reflexes)
- ataxic staggering gait.

Three partners were called into the consulting room to give their opinion. All agreed that Craig's illness was a neurological emergency, although the specific diagnosis was puzzling. He was referred to a children's hospital.

Diagnosis

The admitting officer promptly phoned the news that Craig had acute alcoholic intoxication, diagnosed simply by the appropriate use of the sense of smell. Apparently, Craig and a young friend decided to celebrate the festive season by sampling a considerable quantity of Moselle from a flagon in the friend's refrigerator.

Case 2

Deirdre P, aged 6, was brought by her parents for a second opinion, while I was a locum tenens in a remote practice. Deirdre had experienced 'dizzy' spells over the past nine months and was now complaining of headaches and repeated vomiting, especially in the morning.

She had been in hospital twice and the conclusion was that she had a severe type of migraine caused by emotional disturbances at home and school. Her parents claimed the child had undergone a change in personality.

Significant findings on examination were:

- a sick child with a wan expression
- stumbling gait

- nystagmus
- hypotonia
- uncoordination of movements (finger-to-nose test)
- high-pitched percussion note of the skull
- papilloedema.

Diagnosis

The child was referred to a children's hospital where a medulloblastoma 'the size of a tennis ball' was excised from her posterior fossa. There was widespread local dissemination of the tumour, requiring treatment with radiotherapy and cytotoxic drugs.

DISCUSSION AND LESSONS LEARNED

- Regarding Case 1, why did we miss the obvious (especially at Christmas)?
  1. We did not smell his breath. Even the basic rule of examining his ocular fundus would have paid dividends.
  2. We were misled by the mother's very angry reaction to my casual observation, 'He looks drunk'.
  3. We were preoccupied with the belief that we had stumbled across some exotic neurological catastrophe.

     Remember that some patients with acute alcoholic intoxication (including those in coma) do not have an alcoholic breath: a blood alcohol estimation may be necessary.
- Regarding Case 2, significant neurological symptoms have to be taken very seriously in children. The triad of dizziness, headache and vomiting equals medulloblastoma until proved otherwise.

The incessant febrile convulsion

Prue L, aged 2 years, was rushed into the office with a febrile convulsion, which had been in progress for at least five minutes. The sick child was cyanosed and the convulsion showed no sign of spontaneous resolution.

I decided to administer 2.5 mg of intravenous diazepam but could not find a suitable accessible vein in this obese child. I suddenly recalled a discussion on such a case in a recent update course where it was recommended to administer twice the dose rectally. Consequently, I mixed 5 mg of diazepam solution (1 mL) with 5 mL of normal saline, inserted the nozzle of the syringe into the child's rectum and squirted in the solution. It was such a simple procedure and so effective.

DISCUSSION AND LESSONS LEARNED

- Keep up to date and be prepared for all such emergencies. I tend to enrol for update courses that are relevant and practical.
- Febrile convulsions are a very distressing emergency and intravenous injections are very difficult to administer in children. Rectal 'injection' is simple and effective, and so it is worth inquiring about rectal diazepam injection kits and having them on hand.
- It is important to reassure the parents that the convulsion will have no serious long-term effects and that the child is not likely to have epilepsy (should the question be asked).

Ingesting lethal iron tablets: but how many?

Paul, aged 20 months, was the usual mischievous child who, like any self-respecting child of that age, loved exploring his environment and the taste of lollies. The observant boy noticed that mother's iron tablets (ferrous sulphate) looked very enticing and so, climbing on the table, he reached the bottle in the cupboard and helped himself to some of the contents (a bottle that originally contained 100 tablets).

When he was discovered by his mother, there were several tablets spilt on the floor and the exact number of ingested tablets was unknown. Having read in the medical literature that 'iron' tablets were radio-opaque we quickly organised an X-ray of his abdomen. Paul, who looked as fit as could be, wondered what all the fuss was about.

Outcome

The radiograph was most revealing—20 tablets in the stomach. This was certainly in excess of the minimum lethal dosage (six to eight tablets). We performed gastric lavage. Activated charcoal was not administered because it is considered ineffective for ferrous sulphate. We repeated the radiograph— two tablets remained. Because Paul seemed to be developing toxic effects with tachycardia and drowsiness, intravenous desferrioxamine was given to chelate free iron. Paul settled and made an uneventful recovery.

DISCUSSION AND LESSONS LEARNED

- It is important to have an action plan for ingestion of toxic substances in children. At least having a ready reference in the office and emergency room is vital. If the appropriate antidotes are unavailable or out of date, catastrophes can occur in such circumstances. The author has been caught with outdated drugs (rarely used in the doctor's bag).
- Knowing the various nuances of treating drug ingestion is important—in this case being aware that iron tablets are radio-opaque.
- Note: Modern guidelines for accidental poisoning in children are 'Emesis, gastric lavage and charcoal are not routinely recommended and are best given on the advice of a poisons information centre'.
- We have a stand-by list of the drugs that are very toxic to children; included are anticonvulsants, antidepressants, anxiolytics, analgesics (especially paracetamol and aspirin), digoxin, Lomotil, iron tablets and quinine.
- The importance of packing in blister packs or having safety tops to bottles is highlighted. Since this drama several years ago the packaging of drugs has considerably alleviated this concern.

Nightmare on paper only

The presenting problem

George, the second child of four children, seemed a normal healthy 3-year-old when his mother presented him for assessment. He casually loitered around my office inspecting the medical paraphernalia as his very anxious and tired mother explained their problem.

For about three months George had been having nightmares, episodes that fractured the entire household. His mother, Mary, was absolutely frustrated by his nocturnal behaviour and said she was 'at her wit's end'. She was a small wiry lady who emigrated from Greece as a child. As she excitedly rattled off details of the family dilemma, I noted that she was intense and rather domineering but obviously a very conscientious and dutiful mother. She would interrupt her rapid-fire, one-sided communication to remind the inquisitive George not to fiddle with the doctor's possessions—rather like a vixen snapping at one of her cubs.

She explained that George would wake her at night calling out to her because of a monster in his room or outside his window. She had no idea about any causes for this problem and explained that 'our household is very normal—no problems really'. She said George's behaviour was otherwise normal and he was a healthy boy. However, she wondered if the problem was related to the 'second child' factor!

Identifying the monster

I then asked George about his problem but could only elicit very scant information. Recalling the immense value of the 'draw a dream' (Tonge, 1983) strategy, I asked him to draw the monster. George quickly drew the 'monster' as shown (Figure 18.3). I then asked him about the monster and finally confronted him with: 'Do you know who or what the monster is?'

'Mum,' replied George, very matter-of-factly.

Picking up the pieces

A shocked Mary looked unbelievingly at George and, for once, seemed stuck for words. Realising the delicacy of the situation, I asked George to

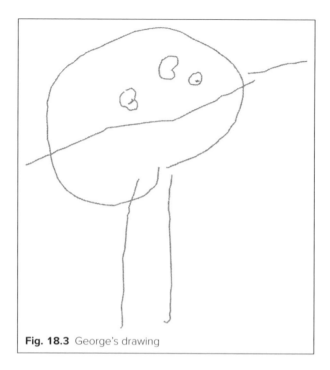

Fig. 18.3 George's drawing

tell me what it was about his mother that worried him. He offered the very revealing information: 'I don't think that she loves me. She's always yelling at me'.

I then asked George if he really wanted his mother to love him. The atmosphere was very electric, touching and emotional as he wept and nodded with a very reassuring affirmative.

Counselling

After some interaction the discussion was manoeuvred in such a way that both mother and son obtained insight that the monster in the nightmares was not really his mother but represented the fear of loss of his mother. The monster was George's insecurity. George stated that he did love his mother and was 'scared' of losing her love. He could not understand why she seemed to be angry with him so often.

I then asked Mary to tell George what things about him made her angry. The resultant interchange between the couple was quite delightful, especially the responses of a very mellow and concerned mother. One could sense that the relationship would be good and the problem would be solved because the foundation was right. The caring was there, albeit misplaced. It was simply a matter of two strong-minded, intense people getting caught up with the pressures of living.

Mary was advised to develop a more relaxed relationship with George, organise some fun things together and avoid screaming at him.

DISCUSSION AND LESSONS LEARNED

- Look close to home for any significant behaviour disorder or other psychological problem. It is important to explore the relationship that is most meaningful to the affected person; for example, husband–wife, mother–daughter, father–son, student–teacher.
- For children with behavioural disorders, ask them to 'draw a dream' especially if bad dreams are a feature of their problem. Key information is invariably revealed.
- Avoid using the old myths and labels such as 'the second child problem'. The author learned the hard way when his second child, at the age of 9, tried to rationalise her unconventional behaviour with the statement: 'I suffer from the second child syndrome'.
- General practitioners can find counselling patients, especially families, a rewarding learning experience. It is relatively easy and is based on sound common sense. We tend to 'hide our light under a bushel' and pass counselling, if perceived as complex, to the 'long stop'. In counselling families we should manipulate the discussion to allow patients to see the cause of the problem and to find the solutions themselves. We are only facilitators and cannot solve the problems on our own.

Children with abnormal features

One of the most frustrating aspects of my early career was an inability to diagnose puzzling developmental abnormalities in children. As a medical student I can recall to my everlasting shame referring to FLKs (funny looking kids). Upon commencing rural practice parents would ask me to evaluate and diagnose their 'different' children or young adults. I could recognise syndromes such as Klinefelter, Marfan and fetal alcohol. However, two young men in particular with a history of poor school performance and learning difficulties, but who were managing to cope with protective family support, baffled me and their paediatricians.

Colin was an obese 20-year-old knock-about who presented with his mother because of his obesity and an incident in which he visited Melbourne and paid for a prostitute to visit his hotel room and pose naked for 30 minutes. No body contact occurred. His mother said that he had an IQ of about 75. On examination the only abnormal features were his short stature, obesity (BMI 35) and small genitalia. Managing his obesity was difficult since he had a great appetite. Mother was not impressed that we could not provide a diagnosis or even a treatment that would make him 'normal'. Of course we learned in time that Colin had Prader–Willi syndrome.

Kevin was a 26-year-old farm hand who had a similar schooling history to Colin, with intellectual disability but no other neurological disorders or physical malformations. Like Colin he had impaired social interaction. He did have features of autism and on closer examination he had prominent ears, a long face and, unlike Colin, had macroorchidism. Kevin in fact had Fragile X syndrome, which is the most common inherited cause of developmental disability. DNA testing is now available to confirm diagnosis.

DISCUSSION AND LESSONS LEARNED

- Forty-three years ago I was ignorant of the above and other causes of developmental disability. We now have excellent disability and genetic services available and referral as early as possible upon suspicion of one of the syndromes is very important.
- It should be emphasised that there is a variable spectrum of characteristic features—especially for Fragile X syndrome—and this makes detection difficult in some cases. Diagnosis has important implications for genetic counselling.

Growing old

The rejected patient who was 'robbed' by her doctor

In early days of country practice I was approached by Tricia, who was concerned about her 67-year-old mother Linda, who lived alone in a small settlement. The problem was that Linda was unpopular and isolated because of her sharp tongue and irrational behaviour. Her husband had decamped years ago and her son-in-law refused to visit her. A recent concern was her forgetfulness and tendency to misplace valuable items such as money. She also had an altercation with her neighbours whom she claimed were interfering with her 'chooks' and stealing eggs—a claim that was denied. I agreed to call on her on my bimonthly bush rounds to monitor her mental health and medication compliance. My predecessor had noted that her 'odd' behaviour was probably caused by fluctuating blood sugar levels because of her diabetes.

I found Linda to be very pleasant and interesting. She was delighted to have her doctor visit her and I looked forward to getting to know this once talented and productive woman. I conducted a mental state examination and psychiatric assessment which was borderline for dysfunction. She complained that her son-in-law was plotting to turn her daughter against her.

Soon rumours started circulating that I was stealing her money during home visits. This distressing allegation led me to reassure Tricia that it was not fact and possibly a delusion. I then diplomatically confronted Linda about the issue and she denied the allegations but said that someone was stealing the money and I was the only regular visitor. About this time I heard a talk that said that this type of paranoid delusionary behaviour in the postmenopausal period of females was called paraphrenia, which is considered to be an early stage of schizophrenia. So that made sense and following her death from ketoacidosis some eight years later (when she decided to cease her insulin), Tricia found a treasured pile of money in a disused stove.

DISCUSSION AND LESSONS LEARNED

- Paraphrenia or late-onset schizophrenia is uncommon but GPs need to be aware of the condition to help management, including reassurance of those family members and friends who are affected by the social trauma caused by people with this condition.
- It is important to continue to support and maintain a good doctor–patient relationship with patients with paraphrenia. This includes shared care with a specialist in psychotic behaviour which involves confirmation of the diagnosis. This may involve consideration of early dementia which some authorities consider can present with paraphrenia.

Slowing up: it's just old age . . . or is it?

I had seen Jack only a few times in the past although I regularly attended other patients in the retirement village where he lived. Jack usually saw another doctor in our surgery. It was not until he developed chronic vascular ulcers on his malleoli requiring regular dressings that I came to spend more time with him.

Initially Jack seemed a rather dull 70-year-old, who moved in an irritatingly slow fashion. I often wondered if he was depressed but as the weeks passed I discovered he had a keen sense of humour, although his expressionless face never revealed this to the world. He always carried a walking stick but never seemed to use it, claiming that it was just to 'steady him' when required.

As Jack signed the Medicare form one day he commented on how his writing had changed over the years. I noted that he started the line quite normally, but that his writing was small and illegible by the end of the line. I had noticed how slow he was to start moving and so I inquired about his gait. He claimed he had no problems at all commencing movement but once he got started he was often hard to stop!

I wondered if Jack could be suffering from Parkinson disease but there was no sign of a tremor. I decided to see how he would respond to a small dose of levodopa. I started him on the smallest dose possible, but even on this dose a marked change was evident.

The following week Jack returned for more dressings. He was a changed man. With a face full of expression and no walking stick in hand, I could see a remarkable difference. He needed some convincing about the extent of his improvement—the changes had been so gradual he had not realised all of them. I questioned him about everyday activities, and with surprise he realised the number of things he could now do easily that had been difficult only a week ago. He was less tired, he could brush his teeth without moving his head, he could roll over in bed easily now and he did not have to shuffle if he wished to turn around. The more I asked, the more he discovered he could do. With joy he concluded, 'Doc, you'll have me doing the circular waltz soon!'

As the weeks passed he became more aware of the changes in his life made by the levodopa, and the expression now clearly displayed on his face was enough to convince me that medication had been worthwhile.

DISCUSSION AND LESSONS LEARNED

- The presentation of Parkinson's disease in the older patient is often very different from the classic picture. In *Brain's Diseases of the Nervous System*, a condition called arteriosclerotic parkinsonism is described where 'of the true Parkinsonian symptoms, the expressionless face, bodily attitude, slowness and weakness of movement and festinating gait are

the commonest. Rigidity is often atypical and tremor is rare in these cases'
(*Brain's Diseases of the Nervous System,* 1969).

• A study by Tanner et al. comparing the clinical features of Parkinson
disease in those patients falling one standard deviation outside the mean
age in a clinic sample found that tremor at onset was more common in the
younger cases, although it did still occur in older patients (67 per cent with
disease onset before 55 years compared with 29 per cent with disease
onset after 67 years) (Tanner et al., 1985).

• We are all taught that the hallmarks of Parkinson disease are the
characteristic tremor, rigidity and dyskinesia, but from this example it is
clear that this may not always be the case. Our minds should be open to
the possibility of Parkinson disease presenting without tremor, particularly
in those patients over 65 years and in those who may have evidence of
vascular problems elsewhere.

Decisions, decisions in the elderly

The two Mr Ms were admitted to a local nursing home at the same time from
a nearby town. They had similar names and were friends. Apart from loss of
hearing they were remarkably fit 90 year olds. Mr M1 was said to suffer from
angina and Mr M2 needed a small daily dose of insulin for his diabetes.

Mr M1's chest pain was reported by the nursing staff, and local chest
wall tenderness confirmed an apparent Tietze syndrome. However, he was
seen lying on his bed, obviously quite distressed, after a small amount of
exercise and this led to investigation of his angina. An Hb level of 70 g/L and
further studies confirmed iron deficiency. A question arose about the cause of
probable blood loss. The author, having just read *Medical Choices, Medical
Chances* (Bursztajn et al., 1983), was determined not to 'over investigate' the
situation.

Discussions with several doctors, including GP registrars, indicated
there was an inverse relationship between the intensity with which the

symptomless iron deficiency anaemia should be investigated and the time since graduation. The obvious answer came from one group: 'Ask the patient what he wants'. Mr M1's reply was disconcerting: 'Do whatever helps you, Doc'.

Ultimately, the decision was made to do a barium enema and leave it at that. This investigation revealed diverticular disease and the patient was started on oral iron. Three months later he had no bowel symptoms and his abdomen was normal on palpation, but he was still suffering from angina and the Hb level had increased only slightly.

Mr M1 later had a haematemesis. A hard mass palpable in the epigastrium was diagnosed clinically as a carcinoma of the stomach. Subsequent epigastric pain was relieved by oxycodone hydrochloride suppositories and oral morphine. He requested no medical intervention and died in his sleep two weeks later.

Then Mr M2 reported a mild intermittent pain in his right iliac fossa. An almost casual examination of his abdomen revealed a large sausage-shaped mass over the caecum.

Immediate referral to a surgeon confirmed the clinical diagnosis of a carcinoma. (Hb level was 97 g/L.) While the patient awaited further investigation, the nursing staff thought he had 'dropped his bundle' because he started to vomit. The diabetes might have been out of control. Sixth sense suggested a visit to the nursing home while off duty during the weekend. Mr M2 was found in constant pain, with slight abdominal distension and not looking quite as well as he had two days earlier.

An emergency laparotomy performed that day revealed a carcinoma of the caecum, which had perforated retrocaecally. A hemicolectomy was performed and Mr M2's postoperative course was uneventful. His only complaint was that he could not remember much about the operation.

DISCUSSION AND LESSONS LEARNED

- Apparently insignificant symptoms in otherwise well geriatric patients should be taken seriously.

- Be prepared to discuss the need for investigation with patients no matter how old they are.
- From a medico-legal perspective, a patient (or their substitute decision-maker) needs to give consent before undergoing any medical examination, investigation, procedure or treatment. Patients are entitled to make their own decisions about undergoing medical treatments or procedures and should be given adequate information on which to base those decisions. The aim of obtaining consent should be to enable the patient to determine whether or not to undergo the proposed intervention.
- One of my vivid memories from general practice was being called to visit Audrey, a 98-year-old patient in a nursing home. She was suffering from acute pulmonary oedema which did not settle with intravenous frusemide. While I was trying to decide what to do next, Audrey told me how she dearly wanted to live until she was 100. An ambulance was promptly called and Audrey was treated actively in hospital, returning to the nursing home a few days later. A couple of years later, we all enjoyed her 100th birthday celebration.
- Presentation of serious pathology in elderly patients might not be as straightforward as in younger people. With our ageing population in Australia, geriatric medicine is a discipline with which all general practitioners will have to come to terms.

Medicine by the sackful

Painting a picture

Ted C was a 70-year-old war veteran who played the game 'be in it mate' to its giddy limit. Before Binswanger disease caused some degree of dementia, he learned all the tricks that some veterans use to maximise the generous benefits of the repatriation system for returned servicepersons.

Ted was a really colourful character whom I first encountered when I was a trainee general practitioner in a group general practice run by characters who were more than a match for any comedy company, as evidenced by Ted's medical record. After the initial shock of the encounter I rather looked forward to visits from Ted. You could hear him coming with the characteristic clanking and tinkling of empty medicine bottles and containers in a sack that he carried over his shoulder. He would shuffle into the waiting room, very stooped, an unshaven kindly face and an air of impatience as though he should be seen immediately.

The first encounter

'Here, give me some repeats of these,' he would say, as he emptied the contents of the sack on the desk. Some small consolation was thinking about the poor pharmacist who also had to cope with the pharmaceutical lottery.

'Do you really need all these drugs, Mr C?'

'Of course, especially since I've caught this German disease—must have been in the desert—Tobruk. The Germans were everywhere—damn good soldiers but they passed on their diseases.' Ted was obviously paranoid and I noted that he had spent some time in the regional psychiatric hospital. (My under-the-desk medical text had no reference to old Binswanger and so I was somewhat distracted by the academic curiosity of it all.)

I pulled out his card and noted the following summary in red.

> *This patient has hypertension and early dementia (diagnosed as Binswanger disease). He is prone to episodes of paranoia and delusions but is not known to suffer from all the alleged conditions.*

His therapeutic armory was as follows [written to avoid confusion!]

1.	'Ear drops'	=	Auristillae phenalis Co.
2.	'Light coff'	=	Linctus pholcodine
3.	'Black with cream settlement'	=	Mist gentian alk.
4.	'White for pain'	=	Mist APC
5.	'White medicine for bowels'	=	Agarol

6.	'Rectal depth charges'	=	Glycerin suppositories
7.	'Algerian pile ointment'	=	Algesal (mist pile driver!)
8.	'Head mixture'	=	'Lotio DDT' pot bromide g.10 phenobarb syr aurant m10, aqua menth prep, ad zii
9.	'MSD'	=	Chlotride
10.	'Blood pressure pills, red'	=	Raudixin
11.	'Light bladder mixture'	=	Mist pot citrate & hyoscyamus
12.	'Inhalation'	=	Inhalation benz Co.
13.	'Stomach mixture'	=	Mist gent. alk.
14.	'Patches'	=	Band-Aid plastic strips

Note: Please do not add to the above list unless absolutely necessary, as confusion is already rife. Mixtures are renamed from time to time as their purpose varies. As all are consumed together, there does not seem to be any case for increasing the variety of medications.

Disastrous decisions

The young idealist agreed that any additions to the list would be bad medicine, but culling the list would be good medicine. Items 1, 2, 3, 6, 7, 8, 13 and 14 were dutifully not prescribed. Ted did not seem to comprehend my explanation that he would not have to swill down so much medicine and would therefore be much better.

The aftermath

Two days later I felt the old 'heartsink' as the unmistakable rattle sounded from the path adjacent to my surgery window. A frantic call from the receptionist led to a confrontation with an agitated Ted, who had 'taken a turn for the worst' following withdrawal of his tried and true 'black with cream settlement', 'Algerian pile ointment', 'stomach mixture' and so on. He did not have many kind words for the new 'German' doctor whom he wanted to 'fix up, good and proper'. He claimed that his system was 'up the spout' and that he would die.

DISCUSSION AND LESSONS LEARNED

- Changing a long-standing treatment plan in patients who seem to be coping with some form of peculiar pharmacological homeostasis can be most unwise. This applies particularly to elderly patients who seem to have a dependence on drugs, even if placebos, which they have been taking for a long time.
- These unorthodox patients should be directed to the same familiar doctor whenever possible and every attempt made to preserve the status quo.

Old-timers and Alzheimer's

One of the most interesting learning experiences of my hospital training was a term as admitting officer in a large psychiatric hospital. I was amazed at the number of difficult problems that would appear under the facade of mental illness. I was also surprised at the vast numbers of severely depressed patients who were admitted as having psychotic problems. Another pitfall was the regular admission of patients with chronic subdural haemorrhage who were sent in as having a psychosis or dementia. Many of these were vagabonds with an alcohol-drinking problem.

Illustrative case

I was called to the home of a 74-year-old man whose wife was most concerned about his health. He had lost interest in caring for himself over the past few weeks. He had become dirty and dishevelled. He was refusing to eat and drink and was prone to urinate in very inappropriate places. He was slow and drowsy, and complained of headaches at various times. Two evenings previously his daughter had taken him to the emergency department of a suburban hospital when he became aggressive and did not recognise her family. After examination the family were told that he had Alzheimer disease and arrangements were made to see a psychogeriatrician.

Diagnosis and outcome

I was not sure about the diagnosis but realised that the rather acute onset was suggestive of an organic cause. There was some evidence that he had a spill from his bicycle prior to the onset of his symptoms. I organised a CT scan and it revealed a right-sided subdural haematoma. He made a startling recovery following craniotomy after a trial of corticosteroids failed to reverse the problem.

DISCUSSION AND LESSONS LEARNED

- Chronic subdural haemorrhage should be considered, especially in the elderly and those with an alcohol problem. A history of preceding trauma which may be trivial provides a pointer to diagnosis but many (20 to 30 per cent) do not give a history of injury.
- The clinical presentation is usually with headaches (which may be absent or fluctuant in severity if present), confusion, drowsiness, changes in personality, slowness, especially in thinking, and memory disturbances. Dementia, seizures or mild hemiparesis may develop.
- A CT scan is an excellent means of detecting the haematoma, but clinical suspicion is the first step in diagnosis.
- Organic causes must first be ruled out before the patient is labelled as having dementia.

Costly waterworks

Theodore, a retired 82-year-old minister of religion, presented to his local doctor with urinary problems. These included reduced force of the urinary stream and nocturia. He was referred to a urologist who, after examination, advised surgery 'as soon as possible before the prostate completely blocked off the urine'. However, since there was a waiting list of 6 to 12 months at the regional hospital, he was advised to become insured for private hospitalisation. Taking the surgeon at his word he proceeded to pay a considerable sum for private insurance.

While waiting to qualify for admission to hospital, Theodore had a transient ischaemic attack and consulted me since his previous general practitioner had left town. Theodore was found to be hypertensive and in mild congestive cardiac failure. I prescribed low-dose aspirin and prazosin.

On review, he happily stated that since the last visit he was 'a new man. My waterworks are terrific—back to normal—my stream is strong and I'm not getting up at night. I don't think I'll need an operation at all'.

DISCUSSION AND LESSONS LEARNED

- It is a mistake to subject the elderly to surgery if other avenues of management are open. This case illustrates the value of using a medication (prazosin) effectively for a problem of mild to moderate severity. Furthermore, it highlights the risk of surgery in an age group prone to cerebrovascular accidents.
- Suggestions to become privately insured often place great financial burdens on the elderly, especially those with limited financial resources. Many hidden costs surface when the patient is hospitalised unless the specialists and the hospitals are prepared to accept the rebate fees. In the author's experience this courtesy is often ignored.
- The general practitioner is the ideal person to offer patients advice about health insurance and to evaluate a consultant's opinion. Such opinions may be inappropriate and sadly are sometimes blurred by hip-pocket motives or zealousness for one's area of professional expertise.

Planning ahead

Mr A was admitted to hospital suffering from septic shock. He was transferred to the intensive care unit where he was intubated, ventilated and commenced on dialysis.

Two weeks after his admission, the hospital staff became aware of a document that Mr A had prepared one year earlier. The document included the notation: 'I refuse dialysis'.

The hospital contacted Mr A's GP for clarification about the document and then made an application to court to determine if this instruction should be followed. The court confirmed that the document was an 'advance care directive' which the hospital was legally obliged to comply with.

DISCUSSION AND LESSONS LEARNED

- Advance care planning is an important part of general practice. GPs are well placed to discuss a patient's future health and personal care where the patient's values, beliefs and preferences are recorded so they can guide decision making at a future time when that person cannot make or communicate their decisions.
- As part of the right to self-determination, a patient can complete an advance care directive that binds a health practitioner who is treating them, even if that directive refuses life-sustaining treatment. Doctors are legally obliged to comply with a valid advance care directive and they risk prosecution if they do not follow the directive.
- The inclusion of advance care directives in the My Health Record will help to ensure these important documents are available when needed.

Chapter 20 — Mysteries of the mind

The challenge of assessing alleged assault

One of the really difficult challenges of rural and remote practice occurs when asked to assist the police in the examination of an alleged assault victim. Invariably the assault is genuine but rarely the victim may present with a bogus claim. This will usually be in the setting of a secondary gain (e.g. financial) but may also occur when the patient has some form of psychiatric illness.

Maddy, aged 17, was brought in by the police with a claim that she was allegedly assaulted by a man with a 'stay-sharp' knife (Kille, 1986; 1991). On examination there was an unusual pattern of superficial wounds on the chest and legs. (Refer to Figure 20.1, centre insert page 8.)

DISCUSSION AND LESSONS LEARNED

- When faced with the responsibility of examination of victims of physical and sexual abuse, it is most appropriate to have basic training in forensic medicine and have the appropriate equipment.
- The account of the assault and examination findings should be carefully documented. Photographs are beneficial. Additionally, the patient's social, family and psychiatric history may be useful in gaining a better understanding of their situation and subsequent management.

- While listening to and noting the victim's claims and providing caring, empathetic support, it is also appropriate to keep an open mind should you have suspicion of behaviour or injuries that are unusual and do not 'add up'. Keep in mind that you may be asked to provide a report on the injuries (only with the patient's consent) and to testify in court.
- The picture of Maddy shows some typical features of injuries that are self-inflicted, namely:
  - all of similar depth
  - (usually) all accessible from the dominant hand (right in this case)
  - avoidance of vital or very sensitive areas such as eyes, mouth, nipples
  - not consistent with the type of weapon used or the fact that she said she was clothed when slashed (no marking on clothing)
  - wounds clustered together in specific body areas with many of the incisions crossing each other
  - no 'defence wounds'.

The man who cried wolf!

Only two months after starting country practice I had a phone call from the local police requesting help in an emergency at a nearby farmhouse. Public servants and a constable had been serving legal documents on a man when he suddenly retreated to the house and began threatening everyone with a shotgun.

The patient

I knew about Jim, a 49-year-old widowed farmer and a legend in the district. A war hero, he was awarded for bravery as a pilot of Lancaster bombers over Germany but in about 1944 he suffered a 'nervous breakdown'. He developed paranoid schizophrenia and with regular exacerbations he spent a total of 12 years in psychiatric institutions. He had been discharged from his most recent committal six months previously on chlorpromazine and benzhexol medication but had not been taking the drugs.

The local community was afraid of him, but he enjoyed the love of his devoted mother who lived on an adjacent farm.

The conflict

Jim had been extremely disturbed when the local dam was built because the state authorities had annexed a considerable portion of his precious dairying farmland. He resisted all attempts at negotiation and his irrational confrontations with government agencies precipitated many admissions to hospital.

The confrontation

As I drove up to the house I could see at the window the silhouette of a very large man with a gun. I was conscious of two neatly dressed public servants hiding behind a shed, obviously disconcerted by the cow dung and turkey excreta adorning their polished shoes. Ruddy-faced Returned and Services League executives peered from behind bales of hay.

Jim became agitated about the policeman despite the fact that he was a genial officer and sympathetic towards him (even though the officer carried some of Jim's shotgun pellets in his anatomy). Finally Jim agreed to see this inexperienced, nervous doctor—alone.

'Give him a knockout shot, Doc, Hollywood style,' whispered the constable. 'Let us know when he's bombed out.'

The agitated and garrulous patient seemed to relax with me. My apprehension eased, but there was no doubt he was mentally ill.

'I don't need any injection, Doc. Give it to those blokes outside: they're Nazi agents. Can you get the prime minister? I'd like to talk to him.'

We chatted aimlessly for about 20 minutes. When I felt I had his trust I drew up a syringe of 100 mg chlorpromazine hydrochloride and shot it into his arm. Minutes passed: no reaction. Half an hour later he was still hyperactive, talking vehemently as he watched for the 'enemy' outside and fiddled with the gun and ammunition he had refused to surrender to me.

He gave me permission to go out and speak to the policeman and I discovered to my delight that reinforcements had arrived. With new instructions, I returned and distracted Jim as a burly policeman crept through the back door to claim him with a crushing bear hug. Jim departed for the long drive to Melbourne, his police escort conveying a 'certificate of recommendation' from me.

Home again

Five months later Jim was discharged from hospital, this time on a massive chlorpromazine regimen. He was warm and friendly but (not surprisingly) rather sedated and dyskinetic.

Knowing he would not continue taking the drugs, I planned to give him fortnightly injections of fluphenazine with the help of the district nurse. The treatment worked well and Jim enjoyed social harmony and an adequate existence on the farm.

'Wolf'

Jim's rehabilitation was not without incident. About three years had passed when the nurse told me she was concerned about Jim: he seemed to be 'high', hallucinating about seeing a wolf in the bush. We possibly had black panthers (escapees from circuses) in the Gippsland bush but not wolves.

I went out to the farm and saw a new and exotic complex of pools: Jim was farming young alpine trout. He was adamant about seeing a great wolf when visiting the trout streams deep in the bush. I went to his mother for an opinion. 'Doctor, I'm so pleased. Jim is just fine. It's wonderful.' Nevertheless I decided to increase his dose of fluphenazine.

One evening about a week later there was an urgent knocking on my back door. There was Jim, looking pleased and a little superior, preparing to drag in the not quite cold corpse of a huge blood-spattered animal, enormous canines protruding from its large skull.

'I got him, Doc! You didn't believe me, did you?'

Although not a wolf, it was a canine species unfamiliar to me and a most eerie sight.

DISCUSSION AND LESSONS LEARNED

- Unfortunately, the family doctor does not have a magic dart gun in his black bag to paralyse or anaesthetise patients in emergencies. Often, agitated psychotic patients are impervious to tranquillising injections, and intravenous medications are virtually impossible to administer under such conditions.

  Note: The depot antipsychotic fluphenazine has now been superseded or is no longer available; another depot preparation, such as flupenthixole decanoate, can be used as an alternative.

- There is no point in being a dead 'hero': be accompanied by a police officer in situations like this.

- Prevention is best. The general practitioner should get to know the labile psychotic patients in the practice and earn their confidence and respect. It is naive to trust them to take their medication. Routine injections ensure compliance and allow better surveillance of the patient. The assistance of appropriate paramedical personnel is helpful.

- Mistakes can be made in the assessment of psychiatric patients and the opinions of relatives can be a sensitive 'barometer' of their normality.

- Many feral dogs and cats roam remote parts of the Australian bush but they are not rabid. Generally, they are shy and can be mistaken in a fleeting glimpse for more exotic, wild animals.

No lead in his pencil

A 65-year-old retired farmer used to see me occasionally with a multitude of complaints: most of them caused by his psychosis. He had suffered from bipolar disorder for many years, taking Parnate and lithium carbonate. In his manic phases often he would stop all medication—to the detriment of his precarious equanimity. His wife had left him; he was desolate and became unkempt and thin.

One time he complained of shoulder pains and some vague chest pains and said as usual that he could not understand why his wife would not come back to him. He had begged her and offered to make the house more comfortable. (He had recently been in trouble with the shire health surveyor for slaughtering sheep in his backyard and hawking the carcases around the town. His neighbours had complained.)

I listened impatiently to his rambling complaints, hoping that soon he would ask for a repeat of his tablets and go. Then he said that he had trouble passing water and had to get up every hour at night, but over a year ago he had fixed it with a pencil. Now he was having trouble again.

I glanced back through his history to find that I had felt his prostate two years previously and had noted that it was soft and not enlarged, and that the urethral groove was not filled in. Recently, he had been taken off his Parnate by an assistant and prescribed imipramine.

I repeated the rectal examination, confirming the previous findings. I said to him as he was getting dressed: 'What did you mean when you said you fixed it with a pencil?' He replied 'I put a pencil in it.'

It was up on the couch again and I could feel a hard, 3 cm area along the distal urethra—the pencil.

The next day in theatre under a general anaesthetic a urethrotomy produced a lead pencil 'sans lead'. (Refer to Figure 20.2, centre insert page 8.)

Concretions had narrowed but not completely blocked the lumen of his improvised irrigation regulator. After the catheter had been removed three days later he regained micturition and I have not seen him since for review. A very sad case and I felt very sorry for him.

DISCUSSION AND LESSONS LEARNED

- The bizarre remarks of psychotic patients should not always be dismissed as symptoms of their psychosis.
- On the other hand, had the patient's wife not left him and had there been lead in his pencil, he would not have tolerated the intrusion for so long.

Lung cancer and the de facto issue

Kevin C, a 49-year-old carpenter, presented with multiple problems, including weakness, malaise, weight loss, headaches, muscular aches and pains, anorexia, shortness of breath and thoracic back pain. X-ray revealed a small pulmonary mass adjacent to T5. Biopsy of this mass was positive for mesothelioma. He visited a city hospital for assessment and subsequently chemotherapy. He was discharged to our small hospital, where the course of intravenous chemotherapy was to be continued.

Breaking through the brick wall

Each day I would talk to Kevin about his feelings and his understanding of his problem, but he was evasive, silent and uncommunicative. He continued to be morose and ill and to complain of a deterioration in symptoms. I became weary of not getting through to him, and so one day I entered his room alone, closed the door, sat down beside his bed, looked him directly in the eye and said, 'Look Kevin, this silence is not helping any of us. Something is bothering you—it's time to tell me about it.'

He took a deep breath and said, 'I know I've had it but I am a lost soul. I've been living in sin. I'm not really married to Ruth. Everyone thinks we are but we've been living together with our kids for 26 years.' He went on to say that he came from a strict Catholic family and he felt he had cheated everybody and was doomed when he faced his judge in the next world. This was the big break we wanted. I spent a long time explaining to him that God is a forgiving God and his problem was not really a problem at all. I offered to ring the local priest and explain the situation. He seemed delighted about this approach.

As expected the priest's counselling, reassurance and comfort worked miracles. Within one week Kevin had received the Catholic sacraments of reconciliation, communion, matrimony and anointing of the sick. All in his hospital room.

The change in that terminally ill person was dramatic. It was a pleasure to enter his room and enjoy the enriching interaction that can occur with the dying patient. Fortunately, his general health improved (undoubtedly aided by cessation of cytotoxic therapy) and he was able to return home for four months prior to his inevitable death.

DISCUSSION AND LESSONS LEARNED

- Dying patients can have enormous guilt feelings and it is important for us to explore them and help the patient alleviate such feelings. A feeling of forgiveness is a very powerful, positive emotion in humans.
- As doctors we can never underestimate the therapeutic value of the clergy in the team approach to the sick patient. We should always be prepared to act as an intermediary in this interaction where appropriate. On the other hand, we have to be sensitive to people's private feelings and not be moralistic or pushy.
- Carcinoma of the lung is a multisymptomatic disease that can be a real brain-teaser in its initial presentation, especially if respiratory symptoms are not pronounced.

A certain kind of madness

Which of us, when confronted with the daunting sight of an acutely psychotic person in full flight, has not at least mentally quivered at the knees and felt like turning and running for cover? Those eyes, with that strange all-knowing look, totally suspicious and distrustful, darting from side to side like a restless flycatcher on a winter's afternoon; a daunting sight indeed. The arrival of the doctor brings sighs of relief all round. Lay approaches and secular ammunition seem strangely ineffectual, yet how helpless that doctor feels in such situations. Quiet conversation, logical explanations and advice seem totally unacceptable, but it is the sole responsibility of the doctor to solve the problem—truly a *High Noon* situation. Just as for John Bunyan's pilgrim, so too for the general practitioner: 'Who would true valour see let him come hither' (Bunyan, 1927).

One who, like me, has been fortunate to live and practise in the same district for several years would find it interesting to look back on some of these difficult cases and see how the people, their situations and problems have resolved. Some such cases follow.

Chas

An intelligent 35-year-old bachelor with many talents, especially those associated with the handling and nurturing of plants, Chas loved classical music. Unfortunately, he had a severe personality disorder, with associated depression as well as alcohol and drug dependence.

His dramatic episode was a violent confrontation with his brother and devoted mother. The attendant doctor was summoned to a barrage of missiles, namely the entire record collection, one by one, and eventually the record player itself; all this in a neat house with a perfect garden and furniture that was cared for.

The next day Chas was persuaded to have psychiatric treatment in hospital. His life over the years thereafter was a series of highs and lows and in one of the lows he took a drug overdose with fatal result.

Mrs S

She was a lonely widow with few friends and no job, living in a dingy flat with dull and drab furniture.

This time the projectiles were cups, saucers and cigarettes, as Mrs S stood unkempt, like a true poltergeist spirit, in the corner of uncared-for surroundings. The same day she was persuaded to enter hospital for treatment for her 'nervous condition'.

After a few admissions she settled on long-term phenothiazines into a zombie-like state. After two major strokes and relative paraplegia, she lives friendless and penniless in a nursing home.

Liz

Liz was a hugely obese, highly intelligent ex-schoolteacher. She was in her mid-20s and had married Tim, a young local farmer who was quiet, introspective, flat of affect, with mild schizophrenia.

They managed to conceive a son who was delivered at Easter. The hospital staff noticed then that Liz was a bit 'high' but paid no great attention to it. On returning home the acute psychotic episode erupted: the combination of the historic religious Easter happenings and a 'message' that the world was coming to an end guided Liz's mind towards the thought of sacrificing a newborn son (and his parents). With the help of our local clinic sister, Methodist minister, general practitioner and eventually the police, the baby was removed from Liz and she was 'persuaded' to go to the nearby psychiatric unit.

Liz improved sufficiently to be sent home, alas prematurely as she tried to suicide by overdose and cut wrists. This time the general practitioner was successful in arranging voluntary admission.

Some months later we were summoned by the shattered husband because Liz had 'gone high' again. We arrived to see her cavorting naked in front of open door and windows to loud pop music, throwing furniture out of the upstairs window to crash down on the garden below. Inside, the house was a mess with graffiti everywhere, smutty and religious; the bathroom door was drawn on from top to bottom. Again she was slowly persuaded to dress and prepare for voluntary readmission.

Years later the (to date) happy ending is comforting. Now, with two children (no puerperal psychosis after the second), Liz is sensible, has good insight, requires no treatment and copes well while studying for an extracurricular high-level degree in education. She remains extremely obese but she has managed to lose an amount of weight by diet and gastric stapling. Is the psychotic volcano extinct or only temporarily quiescent?

Sid

Sid, a man in his 50s, presented one hot, dull, sultry morning in an acute manic state. He was restless, voluble (with unsavoury language), paranoid and looked positively menacing. The episode began in the middle of a busy surgery day and ended at the exit of the premises for all to see. Police help was slow in arriving and counselling was of no avail; eventually, with the help of the tardy officers of the law, he was restrained physically by five people and succumbed slowly to intravenous sedation. His admission to the psychiatric unit was involuntary.

Despite medication, Sid continues to have his ups and downs with bipolar disorder. In the ups he has expensive, expansive, high-flying ideas; in the downs he goes back to the psychiatric unit. His wife aged by 10 years within 12 months.

Mrs K

This woman, mother of two boys, had a poor psychiatric family history but managed rather well, if slightly anxiously, until the children reached school age. Then she became actively psychotic with paranoid ideas about her husband, thought disorders and finally a fixation on her general practitioner, expecting him to look after her completely. When disallowed from seeing him because of the embarrassment and upheaval she caused, Mrs K bombarded her general practitioner with strange and suggestive letters.

Mrs K's illness remains ongoing. Her family disintegrated, she is the centre of a 'committee of care' (social workers, GP, school authorities), and a menacing presence to her relatives, the new medical attendant and the community.

After another violent episode, Mrs K was taken involuntarily to the neuro-psychiatric unit. Mrs K was discharged and is still within the same community. She lives some sort of existence with relatives in a caravan—acceptable only if she agrees to regular phenothiazine injections.

DISCUSSION AND LESSONS LEARNED

- As general practitioners, what have we to offer such unfortunate people? They are so difficult to handle in the acute stage of their illness and we do not know what triggers the acute crises. Specialist psychiatric help is often difficult to obtain, treatment by force is usually necessary and long-term results are often disappointing.
- The cases described here are only a few examples from a large number; it is not an uncommon problem.
- As general practitioners, psychiatrists and caring communities we have a lot to learn.

Challenging drugs of dependence

Lukas, a 38-year-old labourer, presented at the end of the day when most of the practice staff had finished work. He had not attended the practice before and said he was visiting from interstate.

Lukas reported he had left his medications at home. He provided the GP with a list of his medications which included oxycodone 80 mg BD. When asked by the GP why he was on opioids, Lukas stated he had recently had back surgery and showed the GP a scar on his back. Lukas provided the GP with a letter from a Pain Clinic which included oxycodone as one of his medications.

The GP expressed reservations about prescribing Schedule 8 medications because Lukas was not known to the practice. The GP said he would like to contact his regular GP or Pain Clinic before providing a prescription for oxycodone.

The patient became angry and abusive. He said he would complain to the Medical Board and sue the GP if he suffered from any adverse effects from the sudden withdrawal of his medications.

DISCUSSION AND LESSONS LEARNED

- Misuse of drugs of dependence is a major threat to public health.
- Prescribed opioids are regularly sold on the 'black market' and one tablet may be worth more than $100.
- It is a legal requirement for GPs to obtain an authority/permit/approval from the health department before prescribing a Schedule 8 medicine to a drug-dependent person.
- The introduction of real-time prescription monitoring will assist in reducing some of the harms from Schedule 8 medicines and other drugs of dependence.
- Mastering the art of saying no to a patient is one of the most valuable skills for a GP to reduce their medico-legal risk.

Some 'sort of vascular phenomenon'

The story

Betty, a patient new to the practice, was an obese 49-year-old non-smoker who ran a local block of holiday units with her husband. Her presenting complaint was 'I haven't felt right for a long time'.

She proved to be a very unsatisfactory historian. It was a trial even to elicit that the message she was trying to convey was that she was listless, anergic and had trouble managing her usual duties. She answered most questions with clichés or non-sequiturs and when I gently challenged her about this she simply said that she had never been a good talker. Eventually I extracted that what concerned her most was that when watching television she occasionally saw a bluish tinge on the screen.

On examination, the only positive findings apart from her obesity were a blood pressure of 170/90 and a urine test of one plus protein. There was no cardiomegaly, her peripheral circulation was normal, there were no carotid bruits, and ocular and central nervous system examinations appeared normal. I arranged a battery of tests including chest X-ray, ECG, full blood count-erythrocyte sedimentation rate, renal function, serum lipids, electrolytes and MCU and arranged to review her 10 days later.

Her husband brought her back in five days. She had become agitated and confused and was complaining of a severe headache. Her blood pressure on this occasion was 170/100 and I admitted her to the local private hospital. Her headache settled without treatment and her blood pressure came rapidly under control on metoprolol and prazosin. She became more lucid, but appeared to have particular difficulty finding words—and she left sentences half finished. The results of the tests I had ordered were all normal so my working diagnosis was dysphasia secondary to a cerebrovascular accident.

The referral merry-go-round

In view of her age and the modest elevation in her blood pressure, I referred her to the local physician for his opinion. Over the next two or three months, I received periodic update letters on Betty's 'progress' but saw neither hide nor hair of her.

Serums 'everything-in-the-world-you-could-imagine' were duly ordered and found to be normal. The local radiologist got his share with ostensibly normal chest X-rays as well as an intravenous pyelogram and CT brain scan.

Trials of six anti-hypertensive drugs alone or in combination normalised her blood pressure but failed to remove the bluish lights that she now saw every time she watched television. Nor did they overcome her lassitude, her inability to initiate activity and her problems with articulation.

She was then referred to a neurosurgeon in Brisbane, who ensured the normality of most of the preceding investigations by repeating them and adding a normal carotid angiogram to the list. I received a copy of the neurosurgeon's letter to the local physician, agreeing with his impression that it most likely was some 'sort of vascular or migrainous phenomenon'.

Just when it seemed Betty was slipping inexorably on to the physician's 'quarterly review till eternity' list, she developed otitis externa and presented to me again. Making light conversation while writing her prescription for ear drops, I asked about her trip to Brisbane. She replied, '*They* think the blue lights are caused by a problem in the blood vessels', with unusual emphasis on 'they'.

Suddenly it hit me like a bolt from the blue. 'Betty, what do you think is causing it?'

'It's the police trying to warn me about the young people in the end unit. The police think they're putting marijuana in the water!'

Haloperidol 5 mg daily dramatically improved her thought disorder and suppressed her paranoid delusions. The blue lights faded and left and she regained her capacity for work.

DISCUSSION AND LESSONS LEARNED

• 'Tunnel vision' can be very hazardous for all concerned. In this case, the correct diagnosis was delayed and the patient put through considerable unnecessary discomfort and inconvenience because all doctors concerned focused solely on the 'red herring' of hypertension and neglected to keep an open mind about alternative diagnoses.

- High-tech radiology and pathology tests will never replace the value of a history taken thoroughly and patiently. Useful early clues were not pursued with the same vigour as the requests for investigations.
- The words of a tutor in medical school years return to me: 'If you're talking to a patient and you get the feeling that if you were just a bit smarter you'd be able to work out what they're talking about, then it's dollars to doughnuts they're schizophrenic'.

It's just not cricket

A GP was called to a Residential Aged Care Facility on Christmas Eve to review Bruce, a 68-year-old retired plumber, whose condition had acutely deteriorated due to likely sepsis. The GP recommended that he go to hospital but Bruce was adamant that he did not want a hospital admission. The GP was concerned that Bruce may die without hospitalisation. He was not sure if Bruce had capacity to make decisions about his health care.

On closer questioning, Bruce was refusing hospital admission because he considered himself 'too strong to die' and he didn't want to miss the Boxing Day Test match.

After reassurance that Bruce would have access to a television in hospital, Bruce agreed to admission.

DISCUSSION AND LESSONS LEARNED

- Capacity is the ability to make and understand information relevant to a decision, and the ability to appreciate the reasonably foreseeable consequences of a decision.
- It is the ability to go through the process itself that is important, not the decision that is made—a doctor may disagree with the patient's decision but this does not equate to a lack of capacity.

- The law presumes that an adult has capacity to make decisions about their health care, but this presumption can be rebutted where the need (and evidence) arises.
- Generally a person with capacity will be able to:
    - understand the facts of the situation
    - understand the main choices available
    - weigh up those choices, including benefits and risks
    - make and communicate the decision
    - understand the ramifications of the decision.
- An adult patient who has capacity can refuse recommended treatment, even if this refusal will result in their death.
- If a patient does not have capacity, a substitute decision-maker will be required, unless it is an emergency situation where it is not practicable to obtain consent.

Chapter 21

Emergencies, home and roadside visits

A shock to the system

Judge not according to the appearance.

John 7:24

Toward the end of the morning surgery, I was asked by the police to inspect and advise on a body 'found in suspicious circumstances'. In due course, I was conveyed in a police car to where the television cameras and the police were waiting.

The background story was that a man had been arrested the day before for driving under the influence of alcohol and while disqualified. He had been released from the watchhouse at 8.30 pm the previous evening to appear at court at 10.00 am. His parting remark had been, 'I will not be appearing in court'. He did not appear, and on going to the house where he lived alone, the police had found him lying still. When I looked I saw him lying prone in a room at the top of the back stairs—four in number—with a pool of blood spreading from under the head. The light was still on from the night before.

After ascertaining that photography was finished and it was clear for me to proceed to examine the body, I proceeded to turn him over to determine the source of bleeding. I did not usually wear gloves to handle bodies, for as I have remarked to various onlookers, 'The incubation period for HIV is such that I didn't have to worry about it'. Next time I wore gloves.

He was a heavy man and a tentative pull at his clothes had little effect. A hand under the shoulder brought some movement and as he rolled over I felt a 'kick' and there were cracks and sparks, something like a Chinese New Year celebration. After the power was turned off at the meter box, I had a closer look. An electric power cord had been partly unravelled and the electric wires connected to each index finger. The cord had been unnoticed where it passed out from under the body—through a door to a high-power point in the next room. The blood came from where he had fallen on his nose.

DISCUSSION AND LESSONS LEARNED
- Be suspicious of the suspicious.
- Always consider safety first in cases of apparent accidental death, suicide, homicide and motor vehicle accidents.
- Secure safety at the site.

A shocking tale

One very cold wintry Sunday we experienced one of those dreaded emergencies when a busload of tourists returning from a trip to the Mt Baw Baw snow resort plunged off the mountain road. Forty-two people from Italy and expatriates were affected and they were transported to our small bush nursing hospital to be managed by two doctors and two nurses. The scene was somewhat chaotic, especially as many could not communicate in English. Most of the patients had relatively minor injuries but some stressed victims who claimed to be 'shocked' took a disproportionate amount of our time. While moving around the cubicles I noticed one woman lying quietly and looking pale. She then received priority attention and was found to have a ruptured spleen.

DISCUSSION AND LESSONS LEARNED
- Triage of multiple accident victims is a special skill and the process can be affected by stressed patients demanding special attention.

- This event reminded me of a similar occurrence in Glasgow, described by Professor Brian McAvoy (personal communication) when a busload of over 40 people was being triaged at a major hospital and several upset people were calling out 'I'm in shock—help me'. The director of the emergency department requesting 'quiet and order' bellowed out, 'All those people suffering from shock stand up'. To the dozen or so standing people he then said, 'now f*** off'.
- Recognising the dangerously ill patient is vitally important so it is critical to move around all patients quickly and set up head injury observations where appropriate. Pay special attention to the patient lying quietly and to those vomiting and anyone looking very pale.
- Emotionally distressed victims still require attention and counselling.

Don't work in the dark!

It was one of those Saturday mornings when every time you should have been locking the front door someone arrived. Important and urgent matters—a repeat prescription, a certificate for home help, the signing of a passport application!

This call was to see a husband with dizzy turns. He lived beyond the usual confines of the practice. 'No, he couldn't come to the surgery . . . Well he's been having them since yesterday afternoon and the doctor who usually sees him said he'd always come.' It sounded like just one more case of that medical dustbin 'inner ear trouble' or what is occasionally, and quite inaccurately, ascribed to Ménière, and for whose existence Messrs May & Baker must be eternally grateful.

His records, meticulously documented, showed that his dominant trouble was backache, allegedly caused by heavy lifting as a sheet metalworker in the business owned by his wife, a condition for which he was (admittedly with some difficulty) claiming workers compensation. The patient and his family were so distracted by issues related to his back problem that the heading to their correspondence looked anything but professional and their bills resembled those that used to come from the grocer.

His most recent treatment, instituted by a teaching hospital surgeon of his own choosing, included the use of TENS—a discipline appearing to lie somewhere between acupuncture and hypnosis—from which the surgeon, as reported in his notes, claimed he was getting 'substantial benefit'.

At the home (a large Italianate sub-mansion) the doorbell echoed through the halls for a considerable number of minutes before being answered by an obviously anxious wife, dimly visible in the entrance, which was shrouded completely by drawn blinds—a situation repeated in the patient's bedroom upstairs.

His story was that his lower thoracic backache had been present for some two to three years. It was intermittent and several consultants were about to press his claim for justice in the workers compensation court. What at first appeared to be a new form of tape recorder turned out to be the TENS instrument, which was demonstrated and which on this occasion had failed to relieve his backache, his dizziness (that was worse when he was erect) or his mild diarrhoea that had started the previous afternoon.

On examination, central abdominal tenderness was the only significant finding—that is, until his blood pressure was found to be 90/70, falling to 80/50 standing. Pulling up the blinds revealed that his olive ethnic complexion was emphasised by pallor and his diarrhoea was black.

As hospital staff never regard admissions late on Saturday afternoons with much enthusiasm, the urgency for his admission was questioned. Wasn't his pallor due to his southern European complexion and weren't southern Europeans always pale, and was his blood pressure really as low as alleged when his admission was sought, because he was normotensive now? These criticisms were to some extent withdrawn in the face of a haemoglobin level of 7.6 and gastroscopy showing a large penetrating ulcer on the back wall of the stomach, not actively bleeding at the time of the examination. Blood and triple therapy relieved his dizziness and his backache as never before—TENS included.

DISCUSSION AND LESSONS LEARNED

- Be wary of making a diagnosis (even a provisional one) from a phone call.
- Always at least cast a glance at all systems of the body—even at home visits.
- Never believe clinical observations except your own.
- Always pull up the blinds.

Home visits: three cautionary tales

Case 1

It was just before the evening surgery. One of those nights when the partner who usually shares it with you has the 'flu' and the previous message your wife had taken (before you arrived home for dinner) said that a child with abdominal pain was coming and would you see the child before the appointments. You hoped that something less dramatic and time consuming than the asthmatic in incipient respiratory failure, who arrived unannounced last week, would not turn up too.

The patient was a boy of 17, well until two days previously when he complained of mild sore throat. He had attended one of the partners and penicillin had been prescribed for tonsillitis. He had not been unduly sick until that morning when he had become restless and, during the afternoon, progressively more drowsy and somewhat disoriented. His father, a distinguished academic, wondered whether his recent failure in annual exams might have contributed to his general affect.

He was very drowsy, uncooperative and afebrile but with a dry tongue and no other abnormal findings apart from mild pharyngitis. There was no neck stiffness, no positive Kernig's and no evidence of drug overdosage or adverse reaction. He had previously been an active, healthy young lad with no history of serious illness.

Standing at the foot of the bed with both of his parents, now joined by a sister or two anxiously quizzical, and the time being 20 minutes past an expected arrival at the surgery, it was obvious that a tentative diagnosis had to be made fairly smartly. Masked bacterial meningitis seemed a good bet, until it suddenly occurred to me that his breathing was a bit more stertorous than one should expect from his level of consciousness. But what really helped the diagnosis were three large, empty lemonade bottles on the bedside table—not the sort we used to get for fourpence with a penny back on the bottle when I was a boy, but these monstrous two litre disposable flasks.

'Has he drunk those three bottles recently?' I asked. 'Doctor, he's been drinking all the afternoon. I can't satisfy him,' replied the mother. Rather unusual for somebody who is apyrexial. There was no family history of diabetes; he had no prior symptoms of thirst, loss of weight or polyuria; he was too uncooperative to get a specimen of urine and I have never been really confident of identifying the smell of new mown hay.

'I've got a young man with diabetic acidosis.'

'Oh yes,' answered the admitting officer, 'a known diabetic I suppose, and I suppose you've tested his urine for ketones.' Under persuasion and somewhat reluctantly, he dispatched an intensive care ambulance with that air of resigned acceptance peculiar to all admitting officers and with 'they'd have a look at him and see what they thought'.

An hour later he rang. 'You were right; he's got a blood sugar of 61.5 with a pH of 6.95 and a pCO_2 of 11. What made you think of it?'

'Lemonade,' I replied, 'bottles of it.'

Case 2

Bottles also clinched the diagnosis in the second patient.

She was 52, recently returned home from a metropolitan hospital whose reputation for management of infectious disease is international and whose ability to make rapid and correct assessments had, more than once, led at least one local practitioner to wonder how his tentative diagnosis could have been so far from the truth.

During the past year the patient had been admitted several times with 'recurrent' infectious hepatitis. Fifty-two is an unusual age for hepatitis of the infective type and frequent relapses are excessively rare. She was deeply jaundiced and had all the features of liver failure, which included spider naevi, gross hepatomegaly and the first really convincing liver flap seen in a clinical lifetime.

Excessive alcohol intake was flatly denied and her husband supported her, both when we were together with the patient and even more strenuously when we withdrew to discuss the diagnosis. The evidence against their statements seemed so strong that I suggested we look for it. Rooms and cupboards were searched, plus under the house and, finally, a very long back garden. Almost on the rear boundary was a shed, literally stacked to the roof with gin bottles. I looked at the husband, he looked at me and, without a trace of hesitation and with what seemed complete conviction, the answer came to my silent inquiry: 'Oh those—she collects them for the Red Cross'. My remark that I was unaware that august society had gone into the bottle-oh business was received as frostily as my look when we first discovered the obvious aetiology.

He, of course, won. His wife died many months later attended by one of the other partners of the practice, and none of the family has seemed to need my diagnostic skills since.

Case 3

Time was when any visit to the home terminated with an invitation to 'use the fresh towel' and a 'new cake of soap, Doctor' while management and treatment—and occasionally diagnosis—were discussed.

The patient apologised—the bathroom was out of action and would I mind using the kitchen. She was 47, had had a cough and fever for two or three days preceded by headache, her temperature was 104.8 °F (40.4 °C, metrication and its machinations had not yet arrived) and she had moist sounds in the chest localised to the right mid-zone.

That winter had seen a small epidemic of what we used to call atypical pneumonia—now known, of course, to be due to mycoplasma which, we all know, is one of the few chest infections in which treatment can be initiated with a reasonable chance that the antibiotic chosen will be the right one. The picture seemed to fit; a prescription was written and arrangements made to visit her the following day. She was too sick to see me out but 'the kitchen's the first door on the right, Doctor'.

A half-dozen or so parrots in their cages—one or two looking somewhat dispirited—are hardly what one expects to find looking up from washing one's hands in a kitchen. I shot back into her bedroom asking how long she had kept parrots and if any had been sick lately. She replied that she sold them at work—a variety store now apparently branching out from its original practice of selling nothing over two and sixpence (about twenty-five cents)—and that she usually brought home the sick ones, two of whom had recently died.

It was the first and only case, confirmed by rising serum titres, of psittacosis I have seen and, subsequently, the least contentious claim for workers compensation in which I have appeared.

DISCUSSION AND LESSONS LEARNED

So, home visits waste time; make for inefficiency, incomplete clinical assessment and delay in diagnosis; and are really only an expensive form of medical care pandering to patients' whims. But, as far as I am aware, the advocates of multiphasic screening have not yet programmed one of their mechanical devices to scan the patient's immediate environment, occasionally to explore beyond it—or to wash its hands!

Urgent calls to the toilet

Some of my most vivid memories of country practice are urgent calls to people who have collapsed in the toilet, some being in those small outhouses. Add the effects of a cold, windy, dark, wet night and the scene is macabre and unforgettable. In hospital, a call to someone who had collapsed on the bedpan often meant sudden death from a pulmonary embolus or myocardial infarction. In the real world, it usually added up to intra-abdominal bleeding, a cerebrovascular accident (CVA) or myocardial infarction (in that order).

Case 1

'Would you come see Alex? He's had stomach pains since dinner and he's just passed out in the toilet.' I arrived to find Alex, a 68-year-old farmer, on the floor looking very pale and moaning with abdominal pain. The tender mass of an abdominal aortic aneurysm (AAA) could be palpated. Alex was fortunate to survive emergency surgery after the insertion of an IV line and a long trip to a major hospital.

Case 2

'Doctor, come quick. Diane has collapsed in the toilet; she hasn't been well for the past hour.' Diane was a 16-year-old shop assistant and as I drove to her home I wondered if she had been a victim of the pandemic of gastroenteritis that had struck the area. However, Diane had a life-threatening problem. Her severe abdominal pain was the result of a ruptured ectopic pregnancy.

Case 3

I was called to see Hans F, aged 57, a new arrival from Germany who had collapsed in a small outside toilet. I arrived to find his wife and daughter unable to reach him as all 125 kg of him was jammed against the door. All this drama on one of those bleak, howling, wet winter nights. I expected to find yet another ruptured AAA, but after we managed to remove the door, I discovered that he had a CVA. He survived only 24 hours.

Case 4

Eric G, a 62-year-old barman, had fainted or felt faint on a few occasions over two days when he sat on the toilet to defecate. He was complaining of mild abdominal pain. When I examined his abdomen there was tenderness and guarding in the epigastrium and centrally. His blood pressure was 100/60 and his pulse 102. I figured that he was bleeding from somewhere, but where? Our visiting gastrointestinal surgeon arranged admission to hospital and concluded that he had peritonitis. At laparotomy, a ruptured hepatoma was found in a cirrhotic liver and this was bleeding slowly into the abdominal cavity.

DISCUSSION AND LESSONS LEARNED

- A house call to someone who has collapsed on the toilet is invariably an urgent call, particularly if associated with abdominal pain. It usually adds up to intra-abdominal bleeding, because this triggers a desire to defecate and the associated Valsalva manoeuvre reduces the compromised venous return to the heart.

- Associated atrial fibrillation in a patient with intense abdominal pain of sudden onset may signify mesenteric artery embolism. In my experience, if parenteral morphine does not relieve severe abdominal pain, three important uncommon causes are probable: mesenteric artery or venous embolism, acute pancreatitis and ruptured AAA.
- It may be appropriate to learn how to quickly remove toilet doors, especially with older folks who have collapsed (and are often dead) in the toilet. Many have a habit of locking the door from the inside.

A black hole and black snakes

It was during a hot afternoon's busy surgery that I received a call from an ambulance officer. 'We've been called out to this bloke who's fallen down an old mine shaft: the rangers reckon he's dead but we're not sure,' he said. 'He's probably been down there for days and he really smells. His legs are broken and some snakes are down there with him. The hole's about 12 m deep, so do you think we should attempt any heroics? Is it worth hauling him up carefully?'

I decided to visit the scene immediately and arrived to find the men hauling the 'body' up the mine shaft (Figure 21.1). Suddenly, two large battered serpents were flung from the hole: red-bellied black snakes (very dead, fortunately). Eventually, a rather tragic sight emerged: the malodorous, distorted unconscious figure of a pale, young man. Incredibly, he was still alive despite having been down the shaft for almost three days. I recognised him as 'David M', a pleasant 20-year-old who suffered from epilepsy; he was an avid gold prospector.

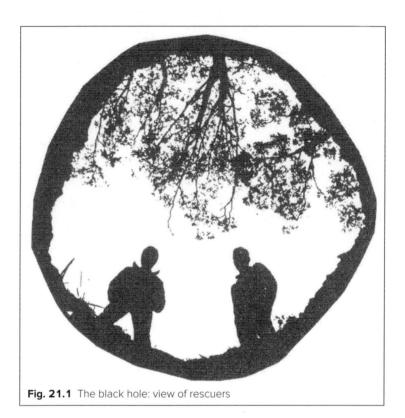

Fig. 21.1 The black hole: view of rescuers

A rapid examination revealed several large lacerations on his scalp and back with a fractured leg and posterior dislocation of his right hip. The foul odour was due to faeces; his pulse was rapid and thready, and his systolic blood pressure was 60 mm Hg. The question remained: did he have envenomation from those black snakes? Red-bellied black snakes are not very venomous, but they still deserve respect. One significant finding really stretched the imagination. Peering into his wound I thought I could see a pulsating artery, but closer inspection revealed it to be large maggots.

I quickly inserted an intravenous line with Hartmann's solution as the ambulance sped off to the bush nursing hospital. David responded to the resuscitation and started moaning with the pain. Cleaning the poor fellow was a task for strong stomachs.

Managing the problem

This difficult case included blood loss, dehydration, a dislocated hip, fractured tibia and fibula, multiple wounds full of maggots and the possibility of snake bite.

The patient's haemoglobin was 60 g/L and so we began a transfusion following typing and cross matching. We decided not to give antivenom but to 'play it by ear'. Removing the maggots proved impossible because of their countless number deep in the wounds (which appeared amazingly clean). I contacted an experienced surgeon who recommended bathing the wounds with chloroform. It worked like magic: the anaesthetised blowfly larvae were flushed out easily.

The patient improved dramatically with a blood transfusion and passed urine that was essentially normal. When he had recovered sufficiently we took him to theatre, reduced the hip and fractured leg, and finished cleaning and suturing the wounds. David made a remarkable recovery, highlighting yet again the amazing recuperative powers of the human body.

DISCUSSION AND LESSONS LEARNED

- It is important for general practitioners to attend the scene of an emergency whenever possible. A request for advice is often a plea to attend.
- Venomous snakes are generally shy and do not bite unless provoked. There was no evidence that David had been bitten despite lying beside the reptiles.
- The lives most readily saved are often those requiring urgent blood or fluid replacement. The importance of performing an effective intravenous cut-down is obvious.
- Multiple trauma are not necessarily as threatening as they appear. A cool, logical approach to management using basic principles invariably leads to a successful outcome.

Collapse in the hairdresser's chair

One Saturday morning while in metropolitan practice I received an urgent call to a nearby lady's hairdressing salon because one of the clients had collapsed. Apparently some minutes beforehand she had been sitting in the chair having a perm when she seemed to fall asleep. She then quietly slid down under the drapes to the floor. I arrived to find an unknown (to our practice) woman of about 40 years lying unconscious but breathing.

One of my first strategies was to perform a blood sugar test by a test strip but I looked in her handbag where a card indicated that she was a type 1 diabetic. This was a hypoglycaemic attack demanding urgent attention. I then had to make a decision whether to give her intravenous 50 per cent dextrose or glucagon, since I always carried both in my emergency doctor's bag. I administered 25 mL of the sticky solution into a good-looking vein and she recovered as expected. This is one of the few times that we can impress onlookers!

DISCUSSION AND LESSONS LEARNED
- 50 per cent glucose/dextrose gives instant effect but can be difficult to give in poor veins and is prone to give phlebitis. The most practical method is to give 1 mL of glucagon by intramuscular injection, followed by a sweet drink or sugar placed in the mouth as the patient becomes alert.
- If the blood sugar is very low—e.g. levels of less than 3 mmol/L—it is advisable to give both IV glucose/dextrose and glucagon.
- Any patient found unconscious should be tested immediately for hypoglycaemia once the airway is secured.

A life-saving drill hole

This tale is a tribute to Dr Gordon Burles, my predecessor at Neerim South, who saved the life of George E, a 42-year-old farmer who was struck on the head by a falling timber beam as he was demolishing a shed.

George had sustained a large laceration to the left side of his head with considerable blood loss and Gordon responded to an urgent home call from George's wife. George was initially unconscious, recovered to a lucid state and then lapsed into unconsciousness on his bed. When the doctor assessed the situation he realised that George had developed an extradural haematoma. He was a long way from expert help and both the local bush nursing and base hospitals.

Gordon searched the toolkit in the workshop and found the brace and bit tool unit. He handed the bit and his scalpel plus forceps, which he carried in his emergency kit, to Joan and asked her to sterilise them in boiling water. He then extended the wound over the scalp haematoma, elevated the visible fractured skull bone and then drilled a hole about 3 cm above the zygomatic arch. The patient did recover and the story is folklore in the district.

DISCUSSION AND LESSONS LEARNED

- It is important for the practitioner working in rural and remote areas, with the accompanying responsibility, to be prepared to undertake an urgent exploratory burr hole for an extradural haematoma. This can apply to other doctors in extraordinary circumstances. I still feel uneasy when remembering that as a registrar I witnessed a road accident patient die of an extradural haematoma probably because the surgeon on duty did not agree with my assessment and also because a trephine kit could not be readily located.

- All hospitals should have an emergency trephine kit available but improvised means of drilling a hole in the skull bone can be used. The old-fashioned brace and bit is fine but the best option is the power drill such as the Black & Decker drill used by Dr Rob Carson at Maryborough hospital in 2009 when he saved the life of a child following a fall from a push bike.

Chapter 22

Lessons in communication

Marriage breaks your heart!

I met Evelyn, a 43-year-old obstetric patient, when I was a medical student. Two of us were asked to conduct a full history and examination with the perennial student attraction being 'an interesting patient with a hole in the heart'. She was great and talked about the straightforward birth of her seventh child and how well her heart continued to cope. Of course we examined her cardiovascular system and assessed her condition as an atrial septal defect. When asked about how her husband felt about having yet another child she replied that she wasn't married but that Terry was the father of all her children. She could sense that we looked bemused and added, 'When I was very young my doctor said that with your heart you should not get married—and I have followed his advice to this day.'

DISCUSSION AND LESSONS LEARNED

This extraordinary story highlights the importance of being careful of what you say and how you say it in giving advice to patients. The days of the authoritarian, all-powerful doctor have long gone, although I guess we have all had experiences of present-day patients hanging onto our words and advice. It adds further support to the importance of providing patient education handouts to supplement the spoken word.

Careful what you say!

Mrs A and Mrs Y were good friends. Each was married with children. The gap in their ages was not great and both had what might be described as artistic and intellectual interests.

Mrs A was a patient of mine. If she came to the surgery, it was nearly always to bring one of her two boys, delightful kids, still at primary school.

After a year or so Mrs A had occasion to see me on her own account. She was deeply distressed. Her husband had announced his intention of leaving her. It was not another woman: it was simply that he felt their marriage was at an end in every practical sense and he wanted his freedom. She felt shocked, hurt and humiliated. The news had come as a bombshell and she had no wish to break up the marriage.

He moved out of the house shortly after this. He would call by arrangement and take the boys out. At other times, to her surprise, she would suddenly hear a key in the front door and he would come in, sit down and blandly suggest that she might like to make him a cup of coffee. While she did not object to his formal outings with the children, these casual 'drop-ins' vexed her greatly. We had a number of long talks in the surgery during which I did what I could to alleviate her distress.

It must have been about three months later that Mrs Y consulted me as a new patient. She reminded me that I had tried to help her friend, Mrs A, and now she wanted to talk to me about a problem in her own marriage. Her husband was being unfaithful to her and she wanted either to break the marriage or to bring him firmly into the fold. It seemed to me she had everything to gain by taking a firm line and I counselled her in this sense.

'Don't make the mistake your friend made,' I suggested. 'Don't let him come and go as he pleases. Change the lock on the door so that he can come and see you only by mutual agreement.' These rather practical remarks were made because she too was being distressed by unexpected encounters with her husband. They were living apart and yet there were some strong elements in their marriage; it seemed to me that successful reunion might be achieved if she 'played it cool' and made a pretence of keeping him at arm's length.

A fortnight later I received a letter from Mrs A. Mrs A's letter was cool and very much to the point. I had broken medical confidentiality by advising Mrs Y not to make 'the same mistake' as Mrs A and she proposed to terminate our professional connection immediately.

DISCUSSION AND LESSONS LEARNED

- My first reaction was to feel chastened. I had been in practice for 20 years and such a complaint had never been levied against me before.
- My second reaction was to protest at the sheer injustice of Mrs A's letter. The two ladies were friends, and had surely discussed every detail of their plight many times over and this husband 'popping-in' problem in particular. I had given practical advice, not revealed anything related to the medical problems of either of them.
- But of course Mrs A was right and I had been guilty as charged. Every GP walks this fine tightrope and it is a difficult balance to maintain.
- Maintaining patient confidentiality and privacy is especially difficult in general practice where we are often treating numerous patients who know one another, as family members, neighbours or friends. Most breaches of confidentiality and privacy occur inadvertently.

Nocturnal spasms

I was woken at 3.00 am by a phone call from a distressed person in the farmhouse of a 67-year-old Italian man who spoke very little English. Apparently, he awoke with the sudden onset of very severe pain in his right leg. The caller said that her father was very seriously ill and would I come immediately. (A 22 km drive into the remote countryside awaited me.)

I made a provisional diagnosis of acute arterial occlusion and sped to the scene. I arrived to find a large household of very excited people communicating mainly in their native Italian. I examined the patient and could find no physical abnormality. He looked perfectly fit and showed no evidence of peripheral arterial or venous obstruction.

Diagnosis and outcome

I realised that the patient had suffered a simple nocturnal cramp. However, the explanation proved difficult and was not accepted by the family group. They scoffed at the diagnosis and argued loudly and excitedly with me. I was very tired and frustrated. He was not a patient of mine and apparently visited a doctor in another town (some 50 km away). I said, 'What do you really expect me to find, or would like me to find?' This provocative statement did not seem to promote a healthy relationship. I departed reassuring everyone that the patient was in good shape. I saw the patient a couple of days later and many times over the next years walking around the town. He was fine but never saw me professionally, and he apparently complained to someone about my attention.

DISCUSSION AND LESSONS LEARNED

- Language and cultural differences certainly create communication problems, making accurate diagnosis and explanations difficult.
- As doctors, we can go out of our way to provide a perfectly satisfactory service for no reward whatsoever and yet receive no thanks, only criticism. On the other hand, we can be showered with gratitude far beyond that which we deserve.
- Common things are common and when I'm called in the middle of the night again for severe leg pain, I will think 'cramp' first but still not dismiss the possibility of arterial obstruction.
- Middle-of-the-night calls, especially when unnecessary and taken advantage of, can make one rather irritable. Such times demand a special, conscious effort to be tactful and not let our professional image down with inappropriate body and verbal language.

A doctor's 'heartburn'

It was old Ben who really diagnosed it—old Ben who spent his days in the customary sloth of all labradors but who, after dinner, went into a frenzy until his nightly walk was assured.

Pain at the back of the pharynx relieved by a good belch after a big meal is surely due to reflux, isn't it? Sure, it occurred on the longish walk uphill returning to the house, but the onset was never quite constant and it seemed to vary a bit with the weather.

So the indigestion disappeared until it was suggested that joining in with Saturday afternoon tennis would mean that we would all see a bit more of each other. It was all right at first, but when my proficiency improved a bit, running for shots after a game or two brought the indigestion back. That, of course, could only be due to reflux after stooping to pick up balls too soon after lunch—perhaps waiting till mid-afternoon would improve things. It didn't, so a good swig of antacid before playing was the obvious answer.

'Ask the chemist for a bottle of Amphojel when you're shopping, will you?' I said.

'What's that for?' asked a suspicious wife—medically qualified but having to deal with the differential diagnosis of chest pain quite a time ago.

'You've brought home 200 mL, but doesn't it come in 500 mL bottles? And isn't it a pharmaceutical benefit?'

'Well, yes; he brought out this enormous bottle, but I knew you'd only take a dose or two as you always do.'

She was wrong—I took three doses to be exact until, a few days later, I met an old colleague who remarked that he had had a bypass since we last met and was no longer in his practice.

I said, 'What sort of symptoms decided you to do something about it?'

He replied, 'Well, I was doing a difficult delivery one night and got this severe central chest pain, which I'd been getting for some time, and I asked the matron to bring me a dose of antacid. I had a medical student with me at the time who looked at me and said, "That's a bit damn silly, isn't it?" and I realised of course that it was.'

So did I—and a friendly physician consulted the next day expressed surprise that what he had usually regarded as reasonable clinical judgement seemed to have slipped a bit. Clinical examination was normal, as was a resting ECG, but stress test showed ST segments sinking before your eyes and before the moving staircase had, so to speak, barely got under way.

The angiogram was fascinating—the quite long narrowing of the left main artery, which remained at about 20 per cent of its usual width in spite of anginine and one or two other manoeuvres, meant that no very strong case could be mounted against 'We'll do you next Friday' when the surgeon pronounced it.

And do me he did. Very efficiently, and with the knowledge that everyone in the unit knew their job superbly, were dedicated and had a record probably second to none in the world.

DISCUSSION AND LESSONS LEARNED

- Never—*ever*—manage thyself. Remember Osler's aphorism: 'A doctor who treats himself has a fool for a patient'.
- 'The diagnosis of angina of effort turns, in a subject of suitable age and sex, almost exclusively upon the history.' So wrote Thomas Lewis in his textbook of cardiology, which was the students' bible in the 1930s (Lewis, 1937). Nothing has changed.
- Various manoeuvres such as belching frequently produce some relief of symptoms. Occasionally one can 'walk through it'. The indigestion often seems less severe during the second set than the first. Cold atmosphere does aggravate it.
- Signs confirmatory of coronary disease are rare.

The case of the odd breast lump

Angela L, aged 38, is a charge nurse who presented for a fourth opinion about a lump in her right breast. She said that she had undergone mammography, which was normal, and had three opinions, with the eventual conclusion that the lump was a lymph node. I could sense that this diagnosis bothered her.

When I examined her breast, including the axillary tail, I could not detect an abnormal lump. When I asked her to identify the lump, she reached high into the axilla and pointed out the 'lump'. It was actually a well-developed subscapularis muscle as it formed its tendon in the upper posterior wall of the axilla. I asked, 'Have you played or do you play a lot of sport?' She replied, 'Yes, tennis, rowing, golf.' 'Well,' I said, 'the lump you have is only a well-developed muscle—subscapularis to be exact.'

She could hardly contain her joy and spontaneously gave me a hug and kiss—most unconventional doctor–patient rapport!

DISCUSSION AND LESSONS LEARNED

- Patients are more concerned and distressed about lumps, especially breast lumps, than we realise.
- Leaving them brooding over a doubtful diagnosis, especially a lymph node, is inappropriate reassurance.
- It is important to know significant anatomical landmarks, especially where important clinical structures are concerned.
- Firm appropriate reassurance for worried patients is a necessary component of the management interview.

Doctor, watch your words

A woman in her late 50s, the widow of a hypertensive obese man who had had bilateral CVAs, presented to a general practitioner with a 'whooshing' sensation suggestive of bruits in her neck.

The first carotid Doppler study suggested an abnormality. This was considered on reflection to be artifactual. A repeat Doppler study and assessment by a vascular surgeon concluded that there was no abnormality. However, in his reassuring doctorly way the vascular surgeon commented to the patient: 'I am a surgeon, I would love to operate on you but I can't'. The patient went away feeling, understandably, that she, like her husband, was also beyond surgery.

She reported back to her general practitioner, who read the report. To be reassuring, he said there was nothing to be done. He also said, 'We don't need to talk about it; we can just forget about it now. Just enjoy life.'

Our patient assumed nothing could be done. She was going to follow the path of her husband. Every night for the past eight years she has put on a clean nightie and arranged her bed. She wanted to be found clean and neat.

Twelve months ago I changed her from oxazepam (Serepax) to diazepam (Valium) and she commented that the noise had gone away. I assumed that she, therefore, felt and agreed that it was a hyperdynamic sensation of anxiety and discussed it no further. It was only when she was in hospital with severe asthma that her story came out. We discussed it that night . . . at length, and carefully.

DISCUSSION AND LESSONS LEARNED

- We try to joke and we try to be reassuring, calm and confident to assist our patients, but sometimes we miss the mark . . . badly. I certainly did. I had looked after this patient for some years, 'treating' her anxiety state without recognising the horror under which she lived.
- Remember the aphorism: 'People may forget what you said or what you did but not how you made them feel'.
- The next day in hospital she looked better and stated that she felt better. However, she had worries . . . her bowels . . . I sat on her bed . . . what was I missing here?

The lovelorn patient

The GP registrar had been seeing Hubert, a 38-year-old public servant, for the management of anxiety and depression. Recently he had started to ask her a lot of questions about her personal life, which she deflected. The GP was worried about Hubert's mental state and possible suicide risk, but he refused any referrals.

One morning Hubert delivered a large bunch of flowers to the practice for the registrar. Although she was concerned and uneasy about the flowers, the registrar did not want to end the doctor–patient relationship because doing so may have impacted on Hubert's mental health.

A few days later, on Valentine's Day, the registrar found a box of chocolates and a card from Hubert on the back doorstep of her home. It was at this point that the registrar realised the doctor–patient relationship must end, and Hubert's care should be handed over to another GP. She sought advice from her medical defence organisation about how to end the doctor–patient relationship. She was assisted in writing a letter to Hubert, explaining that it was in his best interests to seek care from another GP. The letter confirmed that the relationship had always been a professional one, and there was no possibility of a personal relationship.

The registrar handed over Hubert's care to her GP supervisor, who phoned him to ask him to attend a consultation for assessment and ongoing treatment.

Some years later, when the (now) GP was working in another city, she was listening to a radio station which was playing love song dedications. The GP was surprised and upset to hear Hubert asking for a song to be dedicated to her. She was unsure what she was most upset about—that Hubert was still thinking about her, or that the song he chose was one that she absolutely loathed!

Dr Sheilagh Cronin provides another interesting reflection on the challenging problem of lovelorn patients:

> I worked as a solo GP in a small branch practice in a country town in Queensland over 30 years ago. I was treating hypertension in a pleasant married man in his late fifties.
>
> One day to my surprise, he produced a box of chocolates as a thank you for my care. I thought nothing of it until the next consultation when he arrived with another small gift. I said that GPs did not expect gifts from our patients but I started to feel uneasy.
>
> In those days my brother-in-law was working inland as a solo GP and I used to occasionally drive over to locum for a weekend so he could get away with his young family. The drive took about two hours on a very lonely country road—sometimes I would only see one or two cars passing me. Soon after, I drove over to do a weekend and on the way back I dropped in for a morning coffee with a grazier friend on a nearby cattle property.

On the Monday after, my patient came in, seeming agitated. He asked how my trip had gone and I asked him how he knew I had been away. To my consternation and alarm, he told me that he had been worried about me driving on that lonely road and had waited for me at a creek crossing. He had missed me as I had stopped over to see my friend. I knew that if I had encountered him I would have felt frightened as we would have been alone in the middle of nowhere.

I told him that I had been fine and that also he should know that I was leaving the practice in the near future to move to Longreach. He was upset when he left but a few days later he rang me at home to ask me to change my mind. My number wasn't listed as we were living on a family cattle property. At the time I was worried but I felt as I was leaving this would resolve the problem. I felt concerned for him, I did not want him to get into trouble over this episode of transference or fixation on me.

I left and he rang me again once and wrote and then, thankfully, it stopped. The whole experience was disturbing and made me wary of male patients for a while.

When I look back now, older and wiser, and more aware of how the situation could have escalated, I think about what I would say to that young GP.

I would say, talk to an older colleague, don't try and handle it on your own. Maybe talk to your medical defence organisation too.

DISCUSSION AND LESSONS LEARNED

- Doctors may feel responsible for a patient developing feelings towards them, but lovelorn patients may stalk their doctors, either due to delusional beliefs (such as erotomania) or misplaced expectations (often socially inept patients).

- It is useful to seek advice and assistance in ending the doctor–patient relationship in this situation, and ensuring that other practice staff are aware of the circumstances so they do not inadvertently facilitate further contact with the patient.

Dudded by the allies

One day I received a message on my message bank from Fran, one of my regular patients. She said that her medical problem had been finally diagnosed by another practitioner and I could call her if I was interested to know the diagnosis. I recalled that her case had been a really frustrating one. Many weeks earlier I had undertaken a complete assessment on her for atypical chest pain, with negative findings. I had reassured her that she was fine and no coronary artery problem could be found, but when she insisted that she wasn't I referred her to a general physician, Dr K. I assumed from her phone call that he took one cursory look at her and told her exactly what the problem was, making me feel superfluous and irrelevant. With some trepidation, I returned the call.

'Hello Fran, I presume that you are feeling better?'

'Oh, yes. Very much so.'

'What did Dr K say you have?'

'Oh I didn't see Dr K. I went to an acupuncturist, who said that I had a floating rib and sent me to a chiropractor, who put it back in. You should be more aware of floating ribs, Doctor.'

'What next?' I thought to myself, 'Floating anatomy—ribs, kidneys, scapulas, patellas and other unusual conditions such as monkey glands and Texidor stitch.'

All I could say as I composed myself was 'I am so pleased that you are feeling better—that's the important thing'.

DISCUSSION AND LESSONS LEARNED

- Sometimes we are caught off guard by our patients consulting other practitioners who are critical of our management and diagnostic endeavours—sometimes justified, other times inappropriate and mischievous.
- We may feel uneasy about locums who look after our practice. Some are very critical: 'I don't know why your doctor has prescribed that pill for your hypertension—I'm going to give you something better'. I also recall the occasion when a family visited a GP at a holiday resort because their child, Brodie, had a sore throat. The GP was scathing of us for organising a tonsillectomy, claiming that the child was destined for future health issues due to a permanently dysfunctional immune system. The parents had in fact pushed hard for the procedure after eight episodes of pharyngotonsillitis in six months. Ironically, the mother seemed to be persuaded by Dr X. Nevertheless Brodie subsequently enjoyed good health!
- We have to be prepared to admit that there are gaps in our knowledge, especially with unusual conditions such as a 'floating rib', and take steps to learn the real facts about maverick diagnoses.
- It is incumbent upon us not to criticise other colleagues and health professionals for their care, especially with shared patients. Best to be sagacious and diplomatic rather than over defensive.

Chapter 23   Professionalism pitfalls

Twenty years of work as a medico-legal adviser has taught me the following lessons:

1. Good medical practice is your best defence—practice as a doctor, not a lawyer (or as a lawyer thinks you should practice).
2. Knowing when (and how) to say 'no' is one of the most important skills to reduce your medico-legal risk.
3. Every doctor makes mistakes. It is how you deal with these that shows your professionalism. The only real mistake is the one from which we learn nothing.
4. The worst thing you can do when dealing with complaints, claims and disciplinary matters is to be dishonest.
5. You can (and should) always obtain advice and support when dealing with an adverse event or medico-legal issue.
6. Your health and wellbeing is vital to ensure your patients' wellbeing and safety.

Driving dilemmas can drive you up the wall

As illustrated by the following cases, managing a situation where a patient's medical condition means they are no longer fit to drive is not easy, especially when it impacts on a patient's independence or income.

Miss Daisy

Daisy was a fiercely independent, retired lecturer in her 80s. Her mobility had decreased over the years due to chronic back pain and osteoarthritis. Three of her friends had attended the local police station to raise concerns about her fitness to drive. She had been observed to have slow reaction times, would fall asleep easily and did not appear to be in control of her car. Daisy had been informed by all of her treating doctors that she was no longer fit to drive. Her driver's licence was cancelled.

Daisy shopped around to a number of doctors to try to get her licence reinstated. Eventually she persuaded a new GP that she was fit to drive by informing him that she was no longer on opiates and her balance was so good that she was attending twice-weekly dance lessons. The GP issued an unconditional licence, to be reviewed annually. Two weeks later Daisy died in a single car accident.

Bruce

A heavy drinker, smoker and eater, Bruce worked as a long-haul truck driver. He had poorly controlled type 2 diabetes and probable sleep apnoea. Bruce saw his GP for the renewal of his commercial driver's licence. The GP informed Bruce that she was not prepared to renew his licence until his sleep apnoea had been investigated and his diabetes was under better control.

A few months later, Bruce was using his CPAP machine each night, regularly testing his sugars and had his HbA1c under 8 for the first time in years. He told his GP that he'd never felt better!

Rhea

Rhea had just obtained her driver's licence and her first job when she suffered her first epileptic fit. The GP and neurologist both told Rhea that she could not drive for at least six months. Rhea was distraught because she needed her licence for her sales job.

A few weeks later, the GP saw Rhea driving into the car park at the local shopping centre.

DISCUSSION AND LESSONS LEARNED

- Balancing our duty to our patients and our duty to act in the public interest—ensuring public safety and protecting the community from harm—can be challenging.
- The Austroads guidelines outline the roles and responsibilities of doctors in the assessment of patients regarding fitness to drive.
- We have an obligation to give patients clear advice where an illness, condition or injury may affect their safe driving ability.
- Great care should be taken when assessing fitness to drive in situations where the person is not a regular patient, as some drivers will seek to deceive a GP about their medical history and health status, and 'doctor-shop' for a desirable opinion.
- In the Northern Territory and South Australia there is legislation which imposes on health professionals a positive duty to notify the Driver Licensing Authority (DLA) of their belief that a patient is physically or mentally unfit to drive; in other states and territories, legislation provides that health professionals who make a report to the DLA that a patient is unfit to drive are protected from civil and criminal liability.
- Occasionally, when a patient is unable to appreciate the impact of their condition, or take notice of the GP's recommendations due to cognitive impairment, and continues driving despite advice to stop, it may be appropriate for a GP to report their concerns directly to the DLA.

Risky relations

What would you do in these situations?

Case 1

I recently visited my father late on a Saturday evening. He was due to undergo major surgery on the Tuesday. He complained of feeling unwell and having a headache all day. It was apparent that he had herpes zoster ophthalmicus. I wondered if I should provide him with a prescription for antiviral therapy that night, or simply recommend he contact his GP the next morning.

Case 2

Dr J was at a family birthday party when his sister asked him to write a repeat script for some oxycodone for her neck pain. She told him that her GP was on leave and she had run out of tablets. Dr J was aware that his sister had been suffering from pain after a recent motor vehicle accident.

Case 3

Over a three-year period, an experienced GP provided prescriptions to her husband and daughters, including analgesics, antidepressants and other medications. Pharmacists reported concerns about the GP's prescribing to Pharmaceutical Services and a complaint was made to the Medical Board.

A disciplinary investigation ensued and the GP was found guilty of professional misconduct. The tribunal made orders which included a reprimand against the GP, the requirement for a professional mentor for at least 12 months and completion of a medical ethics course.

DISCUSSION AND LESSONS LEARNED

- At some stage every doctor has considered writing or been asked to provide a prescription for a family member or a friend.
- There is no legislation that prevents doctors from prescribing for family and friends, except in South Australia where the law prohibits the prescription of Schedule 8 drugs of dependence to specified family members (unless it is a verifiable emergency).
- Providing medical treatment to someone with whom the doctor has a close personal relationship can affect the doctor's ability to provide good quality care.
- The Medical Board of Australia strongly discourages doctors from providing medical care to family and friends (including prescribing), and there is the possibility of disciplinary action arising from this practice.
- It is worth considering in advance how to refuse a request to provide a prescription, e.g. 'Professional guidelines mean that I am not able to prescribe for family or friends'.

- You can, of course, still be of great assistance to family and friends who are unwell by acting as a well-informed advocate for them, providing support and facilitating the right care from an independent doctor, without taking on that role yourself.

The stripper and the GP

A GP registrar rang for advice about an interesting dilemma.

While working in the local hospital, the registrar was involved in the care of a patient who had undergone a breast augmentation in Thailand. She had suffered from a severe post-operative infection and was hospitalised for intravenous antibiotics.

When she was being discharged from hospital, the patient told the registrar that she was a stripper and invited him to see her at the 'Gentleman's Club'. The patient gave him a card for free entry into the club which he later threw in the bin.

Several months later, the registrar was at a friend's buck's night and visited a strip club. Guess who was there? The former patient who had had the breast augmentation sat on his lap and loudly announced: 'Hello Doc . . . great to see you again'. He wanted to disappear through the cracks in the floor! She tucked a card into his pocket and asked him to contact her. Again, he threw the card away.

His question: did he do the right thing from a medico-legal perspective? If he went out with her and commenced a sexual relationship, would there be any ramifications for his medical registration? Is there anything he needed to worry about (apart from staying away from strip clubs!)?

DISCUSSION AND LESSONS LEARNED

- It is always unethical and unprofessional conduct for a doctor to enter into a sexual relationship with a patient, regardless of whether the patient has consented to the relationship. A sexual relationship between a doctor and a patient is a serious breach of professional boundaries and is likely to result in a doctor losing their medical registration and ability to practice.

- The case presented by the GP registrar involved a former patient. It may also be unethical and unprofessional for a doctor to enter into a sexual relationship with a former patient, especially if this breaches the trust the patient had placed in the doctor.
- Factors that will be taken into account when considering the conduct include:
  - the degree of vulnerability of the patient
  - the extent of the patient's dependence in the doctor–patient relationship
  - the nature and length of the prior professional relationship, e.g. one-off treatment in an emergency or a long-term counselling relationship
  - the context in which the sexual relationship started
  - the time elapsed since the end of the professional relationship.
- Understandably, single GPs who work in small, remote communities may wonder how they will ever be able to establish a personal relationship when they are the GP for everyone in their community.

Looking a gift horse in the mouth

A GP sought assistance from his medical defence organisation about a gift he had received from a patient. The GP had looked after the patient during her prolonged convalescence following surgery for bowel cancer. The reason for the GP's call to his medical defence organisation was that the patient had just given him a ceramic horse figurine as a gift to thank him for his care. The GP was unsure about accepting the gift because:

- it may alter the dynamics of the doctor–patient relationship and create an expectation on the part of the patient for 'special treatment'
- acceptance of the gift may be a breach of his professional obligations
- the ceramic horse was very ugly!

The GP was advised that it would be perfectly reasonable to return the figurine to the patient, and to explain he was unable to accept the gift because it may be in breach of his professional obligations. However, the GP remained concerned about upsetting the patient by returning the gift.

A few weeks later, the GP reported that he had attempted to resolve the situation by offering to pay for the horse! Fortunately, the patient had refused payment and a compromise was reached where the patient decided to donate the horse to the local hospital's charity shop. The GP was happy with the resolution of the matter. He noted, as an aside, that the horse figurine remained in the shop's window.

DISCUSSION AND LESSONS LEARNED

- Acceptance of gifts can adversely influence the doctor–patient relationship and may be an indicator of a boundary transgression.
- The decision whether to accept a gift involves self-reflection and may need discussion with peers.
- It is most important to talk to the patient and emphasise that their medical treatment will be just as good whether gifts are given or not.
- Issues for GPs to consider include:
  - the motivation in the gift giving
  - the monetary value of the gift
  - whether the gift was given during current treatment
  - any vulnerability of the patient
  - the type of gift—personal or generic
  - the frequency of gifts
  - attempts by the doctor to encourage, or to discourage and return the gift.
- If a gift makes you feel uncomfortable, decline it with sensitivity in order to avoid offending or embarrassing the patient, e.g. 'I really appreciate your gesture but our practice policy does not permit us to accept gifts of this value'.

- Medical defence organisations regularly receive requests for advice from GPs about whether or not the GP should accept a gift or bequest from a patient—ranging from gifts of perfume to Porsches and bequests for $500 to $50 000. The code of conduct states that good medical practice involves not encouraging patients to give, lend or bequeath money or gifts that will benefit you directly or indirectly. If you are concerned about a gift or bequest, seek advice from a colleague or your medical defence organisation.

Vaccination error

Ken attended the practice for Q fever vaccination prior to commencing work in the local abattoir. The GP registrar was not familiar with Q fever immunisation and so she discussed the process with her supervisor. The supervisor advised the registrar that she needed to perform a Q fever skin test to see if the patient had had any prior exposure to *Coxiella burnetii*.

The registrar administered the Q fever skin test and asked the patient to attend for review in one week to have the test read.

When the patient returned to the practice, he had significant induration and redness at the injection site, and he also reported quite a severe systemic reaction with fever and headache.

After the patient had left the practice, the registrar discussed the results with her supervisor. It became apparent that the registrar had given an incorrect dose to the patient. She had not realised that she needed to dilute the liquid in the vial and administer a small dose intradermally.

The supervisor immediately sought advice from the government public health unit about how to proceed. The registrar then contacted the patient to explain what had happened. She apologised to the patient for the error and gave him advice about the next steps. The patient was very understanding, saying, 'Doc, I'm grateful you gave me an extra dose'.

DISCUSSION AND LESSONS LEARNED

- Despite our best efforts, we all make mistakes; it is estimated that two errors occur for every 1000 patients seen by a GP.
- Regardless of the outcome of an error for your patient, the following steps are appropriate when managing a mistake:
  - provide and/or organise any immediate medical care for the patient
  - as soon as possible, inform the patient about the error—what occurred, why and how it occurred and what impact the error will have on the patient in the short and long term
  - apologise for the error
  - inform the patient of the steps that will be taken to minimise the possibility of a similar mistake occurring in the future
  - invite any comments and questions from the patient
  - take steps to look after yourself, e.g. discuss with a colleague and/or your medical defence organisation.
- Patients are often incredibly forgiving of errors by their doctors, especially if an honest and open discussion occurs.
- Ensuring a mistake is managed appropriately and professionally is vital for the welfare of our patients—and us.

The importance of being a good Samaritan

One of my most memorable medico-legal calls was from a GP who had managed to safely deliver a premature baby on an international flight.

It was five hours into the flight when the call was made: 'Is there a doctor on board?' The GP's husband, an ophthalmologist, confidently volunteered to attend but quickly returned to get his wife's help.

The patient was lying in the galley with the baby's head in view. In what sounded like an extraordinary feat of teamwork and equipment improvisation, the GP managed to safely deliver the baby and the placenta. The plane was diverted and a well baby and relieved mother were transferred to hospital for ongoing care.

The GP rang on her arrival in London—certainly not a case of medico-legal concern for the GP!

DISCUSSION AND LESSONS LEARNED

- Doctors sometimes express concerns about the possibility of being sued as a result of good Samaritan acts.
- The possibility of legal action arising out of a good Samaritan act is extremely remote and the author is not aware of any claim in Australia involving a good Samaritan doctor's actions. Legislation exists in every Australian state and territory which provides protection from liability for good Samaritans. The purpose of this legislation is to encourage everyone, particularly health professionals, to assist strangers who are in need of medical assistance without the fear of any legal repercussions from an error in treatment.

Chapter 24

Cautionary methods: towards a safe diagnostic strategy

The stories told in this book demand that general practitioners have an incisive, detective-like approach to our discipline, which is arguably the most difficult, complex and challenging of the healing arts. Our field of endeavour is at the very front line of medicine and, as practitioners of first contact, we shoulder the responsibility of the early diagnosis of very serious, perhaps life-threatening, illness in addition to the recognition of anxiety traits in our patients.

Over and over again the old medicine adage 'More things are missed by not looking than by not knowing' has been stressed. However, our area is characterised by a wide kaleidoscope of presenting problems, often foreign to the classic textbook presentation and sometimes embellished by a 'shopping list' of seemingly unconnected problems—the so-called *undifferentiated illness syndrome*. It is important, especially in a busy practice, to adopt a fail-safe strategy to analyse such presenting problems. Such an approach is even more important in a world of increasing medical litigation and specialisation.

It has been estimated that the diagnostic error rate in a general practice setting is 10–15 per cent. Fortunately most of these errors do not cause harm to patients, but some do. Indeed, diagnostic error is the underlying cause of approximately half of the medical negligence claims involving Australian GPs.

For the individual GP, building knowledge and knowledge organisation are important means of reducing diagnostic error. Some of the ways in which to reduce diagnostic errors include:

- building and strengthening the repository of illness scripts
    - knowledge of atypical presentation of diseases
    - symptom-based and case report reading
- 'thinking about your thinking'
    - what else could this be?
    - what finding doesn't fit with my diagnosis?
    - is there any reason to slow down?
- acknowledge emotions
    - external demands
    - internal stresses
    - emotions stemming from patient interactions
- reducing reliance on memory
    - use of checklists, clinical references and/or clinical decision support tools.

To help bring order to the jungle of general practice problems, the author has developed a simple model to facilitate diagnosis and reduce the margin of error.

The basic model

The use of the diagnostic model requires a disciplined approach to the problem, with the medical practitioner having to quickly answer five self-posed questions. The questions, for a particular patient, are as shown in the box on the next page.

This approach, based on considerable experience, requires the learning of a predetermined plan, which naturally would vary in different parts of the world but would have a certain universal application in the so-called developed world.

> **The diagnosis model for a presenting problem**
> **1.** What is the probability diagnosis?
> **2.** What serious disorder(s) must not be missed?
> **3.** What conditions are often missed (the pitfalls)?
> **4.** Could this patient have one of the 'masquerades'?
> **5.** Is this patient trying to tell me something else?

Each of the five questions will be expanded upon.

1. What is the probability diagnosis?

The probability diagnosis is based on the doctor's perspective and experience regarding prevalence, incidence and the natural history of disease. The general practitioner acquires first-hand epidemiological knowledge about the patterns of illness (apparent in individuals and in the community) which enables him or her to view illness from a perspective that is not available to doctors in other disciplines. Thus, during the medical interview, the doctor is not only gathering information, allocating priorities and making hypotheses, but is also developing a probability diagnosis based on acquired epidemiological knowledge.

2. What serious disorder(s) must not be missed?

While epidemiological knowledge is a great asset to the general practitioner, it can be a disadvantage in that what is common is so familiar that the all-important rare cause of a presenting symptom may be overlooked. On the other hand, the doctor in the specialist clinic, where a different spectrum of disease is encountered, is more likely to focus on the rare at the expense of the common cause. However, it is vital, especially working in the modern framework of a litigation-conscious society, not to miss serious, life-threatening disorders.

To achieve early recognition of serious illness the general practitioner needs to develop a 'high index of suspicion'. This is generally regarded as largely intuitive, but this is probably not so, and it would be more accurate to say that it comes with experience.

Serious, not-to-be-missed conditions

- Neoplasia, especially malignancy
- HIV infection
- Severe infection, especially:
    - meningoencephalitis
    - septicaemia
    - *Haemophilus influenzae* type b
    - tuberculosis
    - clostridia infections
    - bacterial endocarditis
- Acute coronary syndromes
    - myocardial infarction
    - unstable angina
    - arrhythmias
- Intracerebral lesions, e.g. subarachnoid haemorrhage
- Severe asthma
- Imminent or potential suicide

The serious disorders that should always be considered 'until proved otherwise' include malignant disease, coronary disease and life-threatening infections such as meningitis, septicaemia and bacterial endocarditis (see the box titled 'Serious, not-to-be-missed conditions').

Acute coronary syndromes, especially myocardial infarction, are extremely important to consider because they are potentially lethal and at times can be overlooked by the busy practitioner. It does not always manifest as the classic presentation of crushing central pain; it can present as pain of varying severity and quality in a wide variety of sites. These sites include the jaw, neck, arm, epigastrium and interscapular region (Figure 24.1).

Coronary artery disease may manifest as life-threatening arrhythmias, which may present as palpitations and/or dizziness. A high index of suspicion is necessary to diagnose arrhythmias.

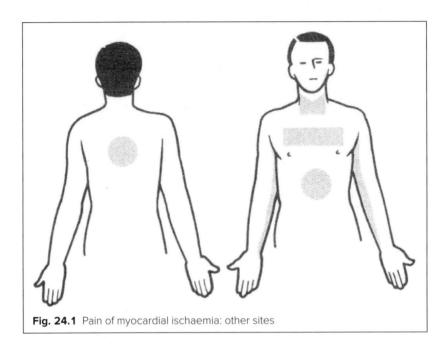

Fig. 24.1 Pain of myocardial ischaemia: other sites

A useful mnemonic for thinking danger is VIC:

- Vascular
- Infection (severe)
- Cancer.

Red flags

Red flags (alarm bells) are symptoms or signs that alert us to the likelihood of significant harm. Examples include weight loss, persistent vomiting, altered cognition, fever >38 °C, dizziness/syncope (especially at the toilet) and pallor.

Think fast with management of infarction

Remember the ideal intervention time rules:

- acute coronary states—60 to 90 minutes
- stroke—cerebral infarct—three to four hours

- femoral artery—four hours
- limb salvage—four hours; more than six hours = limb amputation
- torsion of testes—four to six hours.

3. What conditions are often missed?

This question refers to the common 'pitfalls' so often encountered in general practice. This area is definitely related to the experience factor and includes rather simple non-life-threatening problems that can be so easily overlooked unless doctors are prepared to include them in their diagnostic framework. Examples include smoking or dental caries as a cause of abdominal pain; occupational or environmental hazards as a cause of headache; and faecal impaction as a cause of diarrhoea. We have all experienced the 'red face syndrome' from a urinary tract infection, whether it is the cause of fever in a child, lumbar pain in a pregnant woman or malaise in an older person. Other classic pitfalls include allergies, *Candida albicans* infection, domestic abuse, child abuse, drugs, foreign bodies, early pregnancy, Paget disease, coeliac disease, haemochromatosis, endometriosis, sarcoidosis, faecal impaction, migraine (atypical variants) and seizure disorders.

4. Could this patient have one of the 'masquerades'?

The author sometimes refers to these important problems as the 'sins of omission' in general practice, because the conditions appear to be so often overlooked as the cause of the symptom complex in the patient presenting with undifferentiated illness.

It is important to utilise a type of fail-safe mechanism to avoid missing the diagnosis of these disorders. Some practitioners refer to consultations that make their 'head spin' in confusion and bewilderment with patients presenting with a 'shopping list' of problems. It is for these patients that a checklist is useful. Consider the apparent neurotic patient who presents with headache, lethargy, tiredness, constipation, anorexia, indigestion, shortness of breath on exertion, pruritus, flatulence, sore tongue and backache.

In such a patient we must consider a diagnosis that links all these symptoms, especially if the physical examination is inconclusive, and this includes iron-deficiency anaemia, depression, diabetes mellitus, hypothyroidism or drug abuse.

A century ago it was important to consider diseases such as syphilis and tuberculosis as the great common masquerades, but these infections have been replaced by iatrogenesis, malignant disease, alcoholism, endocrine disorders and the various manifestations of atherosclerosis, particularly coronary insufficiency and cerebrovascular insufficiency.

If the patient has pain anywhere it is possible that it could originate from the spine, and so the possibility of spinal pain (radicular or referred) should be considered as the cause for various pain syndromes such as headache, arm pain, leg pain, chest pain, pelvic pain and even abdominal pain. The author's experience is that spondylogenic pain is one of the most underdiagnosed problems in general practice.

A checklist has been divided into two groups of seven disorders (see the boxes titled 'The seven primary masquerades' and 'The seven other masquerades'). The first list of the primary masquerades represents the more common disorders encountered in general practice; the second list includes less common masquerades, although the latter is more relevant to consultant practice. Some conditions in the second list—such as infectious mononucleosis—can be very common masquerades in general practice. Systemic lupus erythematosus (SLE) is referred to as 'the great pretender'. Likewise coeliac disease can be considered a classic masquerade. Neoplasia, especially of the so-called 'silent areas' can pose an elusive diagnostic problem. Typical examples are carcinoma of the nasopharynx and sinuses, ovary, caecum, kidney and lymphopoietic system. As a practical diagnostic ploy, the author has both lists strategically placed on the surgery wall immediately behind the patient. The lists are rapidly perused for inspiration should the diagnosis for a particular patient prove elusive.

The seven primary masquerades

1. Depression
2. Diabetes mellitus
3. Drugs
   - iatrogenic
   - self-abuse
     - alcohol
     - opioids
     - nicotine
     - others
4. Anaemia
5. Thyroid and other endocrine disorders, e.g.
   - hyperthyroidism
   - hypothyroidism
   - Addison disease
6. Urinary infection
7. Spinal dysfunction

The seven other masquerades

1. Chronic renal failure
2. Malignant disease
   - lymphomas
   - lung
   - caecum/colon
   - kidney
   - multiple myeloma
   - ovary
3. HIV infection
4. Rheumatic disorders
   - polymyalgia rheumatica
   - systemic lupus erythematosus (SLE)
   - rheumatoid arthritis
   - systemic sclerosis
5. Neurological dilemmas
   - Parkinson disease
   - Guillain–Barré syndrome
   - multiple sclerosis
   - seizure disorders
   - migraine and its variants
6. Subacute/chronic infections, e.g.
   - zoonoses
   - tuberculosis
   - infective endocarditis
   - Epstein–Barr virus (EBV) mononucleosis
   - hepatitis (various)
7. Other infections
   - malaria
   - pneumonia, especially atypical pneumonia
   - sexually transmitted infections (STIs), e.g. syphilis

5. Is the patient trying to tell me something else?

The doctor has to consider, especially in the case of undifferentiated illness, whether the patient has a 'hidden agenda' for the presentation. Of course, the patient may be depressed (overt or masked) or may have a true anxiety state. However, a presenting symptom such as tiredness may represent a 'ticket of entry' to the consulting room. It may represent a plea for help in a stressed or anxious patient. We should be sensitive to patients' needs and feelings, and as listening, caring, empathetic practitioners provide the right opportunity for the patient to communicate freely.

Deep sexual anxieties and problems, poor self-esteem, and fear of malignancy or some other medical catastrophe are just some of the reasons patients present to doctors. The author has another checklist titled 'Underlying fears or image problems causing stress and anxiety' to help identify the psychosocial reasons for the patient's malaise.

Underlying fears or image problems causing stress and anxiety
1. Interpersonal conflict in the family
2. Identification with sick or deceased friends
3. STIs, especially HIV
4. Impending 'coronary' or 'stroke'
5. Sexual problem
6. Drug-related problem
7. Fear of malignancy
8. Crippling arthritis
9. Financial woes
10. Other abnormal stressors

In the author's experience of counselling patients and families, the problems caused by interpersonal conflict are quite amazing and make it worthwhile specifically exploring the quality of close relationships, such as the husband–wife, mother–daughter and father–son relationships.

Another common yet overlooked stressor is bullying, whether it is in the workplace, school, tertiary institution, home, internet or elsewhere. It is a significant public health issue. As GPs we should be more aware of the possibility that workplace bullying may be contributing to the presenting illness. A simple, direct routine question such as 'How are things at work?' can create an opportunity to identify the issue.

Identification and transference of illness, symptoms and death, in particular, are important areas of anxiety to consider. Patients often identify their problems with relatives, friends or public personalities who have malignant disease. Other somatoform disorders, including the fascinating Munchausen syndrome (also known as factitious disorder) or Munchausen syndrome by proxy, may be obvious or extremely complex and difficult to recognise. These subtle psychosocial issues are usually referred to as 'yellow flags'.

Some examples of application of the model

Headache

1. Q.   What is the probability diagnosis?
   A.   Tension headache

2. Q.   What serious disorder(s) must not be missed?
   A.   Vascular
   - Subarachnoid haemorrhage
   - Intracerebral haemorrhage
   - Subdural/extradural haematoma
   - Temporal arteritis
   Infection
   - Meningitis
   - Encephalitis
   - Cerebral abscess
   Neoplasia
   - Cancer
   - Benign tumour

3. Q. What conditions are often missed?

A. Cervical spondylosis/dysfunction

Refractive error of eye

Sinusitis

Exertional headache

(and possibly those above under question 2)

4. Q. Could the patient have one of the 'masquerades'?

A.	
Depression	Yes
Diabetes	—
Drugs	Yes
Anaemia	Yes
Thyroid disease	—
Urinary infection	—
Spinal dysfunction	Yes

5. Q. Is this patient trying to tell me something else?

A. Headache is a very common functional symptom and may certainly represent a plea for help for an underlying psychogenic disorder.

Lower back pain

1. Q. What is the probability diagnosis?

A. Vertebral dysfunction (non-specific back pain)

Musculoskeletal strain

Spondylosis (degenerative arthritis)

2. Q. What serious disorder(s) must not be missed?

A. Vascular

- Ruptured aortic retroperitoneal aneurysm
- Retroperitoneal haemorrhage (anticoagulants)

Infection
- Osteomyelitis; TB
- Epidural abscess
- Septic discitis

Cancer
- Myeloma
- Metastases

Vertebral fracture, including osteoporotic fracture

3. Q. What conditions are often missed?

A. Spondyloarthropathies, e.g. ankylosing spondylitis

Reiter's syndrome

Spondylolisthesis

Claudication—vascular or neurogenic

4. Q. Could this patient have one of the 'masquerades'?

A.	
Depression	Yes
Diabetes	—
Drugs	—
Anaemia	—
Thyroid disease	—
Urinary infection	Yes
Spinal dysfunction	Yes

5. Q. Is this patient trying to tell me something else?

A. Quite likely. Consider lifestyle stresses, job dissatisfaction, malingering and conversion reaction.

Index